What Young People Want from Mental Health Services

I0130357

Young people experience one of the highest rates of mental health problems of any group, but make the least use of the support available to them. To reach young people in distress, we need to understand what this digital generation want from mental health professionals and services.

Based on interviews with nearly 400 young people, this book offers a vision of youth mental health issues and services through the eyes of young people themselves. It offers professionals important insights into the meaning of identity and agency for this generation and explores how these issues play out in young people's expectations of mental health support. It shows how, despite young people's immersion in digital technology, genuine and trusting relationships remain a key ingredient in their priorities for support. It considers what access to mental health support means for a generation who have grown up with the immediacy enabled by digital technology. Young people's accounts also provide crucial insights into how they are using digital resources to manage their own mental health — in ways often not appreciated by professionals who design internet interventions.

What Young People Want from Mental Health Services offers clear guidance to counsellors, psychologists, psychiatrists, youth workers, social workers, service providers, and policymakers about how to work with youth and design their services so they are a better match for young people today. It contributes to a growing movement calling for a 'Youth Informed Approach' to mental health to address the needs of young people.

Kerry Gibson is an Associate Professor in the School of Psychology at the University of Auckland. She is a clinical psychologist with extensive experience working with young people. Her research, conducted through *The Mirror Project*, seeks to ensure young people's views are represented in the design of mental health services.

What Young People Want from Mental Health Services

A Youth Informed Approach for the Digital Age

Kerry Gibson

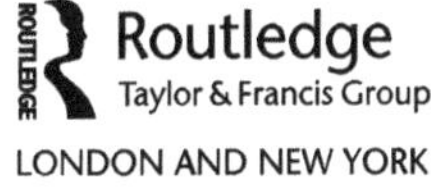

LONDON AND NEW YORK

First published 2022
by Routledge
2 Park Square, Milton Park, Abingdon, Oxon OX14 4RN

and by Routledge
605 Third Avenue, New York, NY 10158

Routledge is an imprint of the Taylor & Francis Group, an informa business

British Library Cataloguing-in-Publication Data
A catalogue record for this book is available from the British Library

Library of Congress Cataloging-in-Publication Data
Names: Gibson, Kerry, author.
Title: What young people want from mental health services : a youth informed approach for the digital age / authored by Kerry Gibson.
Description: First. | Milton Park, Abingdon, Oxon ; New York, NY : Routledge, 2022. | Includes bibliographical references and index. | .
Identifiers: LCCN 2021018904 | ISBN 9780367338589 (hardback) | ISBN 9780367338596 (paperback) | ISBN 9780429322457 (ebook)
Subjects: LCSH: Mental health services. | Mental health policy. | Teenagers.
Classification: LCC RA790.5 .G52 2022 | DDC 362.10835--dc23
LC record available at https://lccn.loc.gov/2021018904

ISBN: 978-0-367-33858-9 (hbk)
ISBN: 978-0-367-33859-6 (pbk)
ISBN: 978-0-429-32245-7 (ebk)

DOI: 10.4324/9780429322457

Typeset in Galliard
by MPS Limited, Dehradun

This book is dedicated to my father, Rex Gibson, who encouraged and inspired me to write it; to my son, James Fox, who has been an invaluable informant on young people; and to my husband, Tom Fox, whose love and support has sustained me through this project.

Contents

Preface

Kerry Gibson

Working as a clinical psychologist, I had an inkling that I was missing something about what my young clients were looking for in their encounters with me and my professional colleagues. When things went well, they thanked me at the end of our time together but sometimes seem to have taken something from the process that I had not been aware of giving. More concerningly, there were times when a young client seemed to lose interest in coming to see me, and too often dropped out of therapy altogether, for reasons I did not altogether understand.

I began to ask my young clients more directly about what they were looking for from me and from other professionals they might have seen during their journey through the mental health system. I had expected them to say that they were hoping for help to deal with their problems or perhaps to feel better about themselves. Instead, they surprised me by talking more about how they wanted to be 'understood' or that they just wanted an opportunity 'to talk.' When they spoke about their counsellors (or psychologists, or psychiatrists) they seldom mentioned their expertise and, in fact, often seemed confused about what these people's professional qualifications had been. Young people rather seemed to comment on how their counsellors had been 'nice,' or 'kind,' or 'had a good sense of humour.' I also heard surprisingly little about their bad experiences with mental health professionals. I found myself drawn by a curiosity about what mattered to young people in their encounters with mental health professionals, what they were looking for, and what they took away from these experiences. I also wondered particularly about what stories my colleagues and I were *not* hearing, and what these might tell us about how to better reach young people experiencing distress.

I began *The Mirror Project* in 2012 with the intention of trying to capture the experience of counselling through the eyes of young people. This was not only sparked by the clinical experiences I describe above but also driven by a combination of urgent concern and helplessness about the high rates of mental health difficulties and suicide among young people in New Zealand and elsewhere. I was particularly aware that young people were making poor use of the mental health services available to them, a fact which suggested some fundamental mismatch between the way these were designed and youth priorities. I wanted to hear more, in young people's own words, about what they were struggling with and how we could help.

My research direction felt at the time like a rather radical departure from the trend in clinical psychology research, which mostly seemed focused on identifying mental health problems and testing out which interventions worked, or did not work, in reducing the severity of symptoms. The idea of simply exploring how young people might experience mental health support seemed a somewhat frivolous pursuit in comparison. But as I continued this work, I became increasingly convinced that young people's accounts of their experiences with mental health professionals could be a rich source of knowledge for those wanting to support them.

Although I considered myself as someone who related well to young people and felt an affinity with their concerns, my conversations with them outside of the therapy room offered a different lens on some of my assumptions. Like many professionals in my generation, I had found myself relying on my own experience of youth to provide a bridge to the young people I worked with. But my eyes were opened to a world that felt quite different to the one that I had experienced in my teens and early 20s. With this realisation, I became more interested in the distinctive social and economic challenges young people were facing today and began to understand how this might influence their experiences of distress and their expectations of help. This broader lens offered insights about *what* young people wanted from mental health support, but also, importantly, an understanding of *why* these things mattered to them.

I was initially not particularly interested in young people's use of digital technology. Although I use digital communication technology in my life, I shared a view common to my generation that textual communication was a second-best way of talking about deeply personal issues. But in spite of my own scepticism about the value of digital communication, the young people I spoke to showed me more clearly what this technology meant to them, and how they were able to use it to talk about things that were very important to them. Recognising the role digital technology played young people's lives also added another layer to my understanding of the social milieu that young people inhabit. I began to see how their immersion in a digital world not only contributed new challenges and opportunities for young people, but also changed the way they saw themselves, others, and their hopes and fears for their future.

I also began to recognise ways in which mental health professionals were approaching young people's use of digital communication — especially social media — might be contributing to a growing gap in understanding between the generations. While I appreciate that there are risks for young people associated with social media, I wanted to move away from this restrictive narrative to better understand how young people themselves engage with these resources especially in relation to seeking help for mental health distress. I believe strongly, that if we want to reach young people experiencing mental health distress, we need to see how we can get alongside them and support them in the digital world that they inhabit.

This book relies heavily on broad strokes to sketch out an understanding of some of the things that young people might struggle with today and what appropriate mental health support might look like. I recognise that in this, there is potential to lose the nuance and heterogeneity of young people's experiences. This book draws almost exclusively from New Zealand data and cannot capture the diversity of people's experiences around the world, but I hope that it has some relevance to countries where the economic and social landscape is similar. I am aware that, as always in research, we tend to capture the voices of those who are willing and able to speak out about their experience. There are other more marginalised voices we tend to hear less of in research, and they might easily be those whose mental health is most vulnerable. It is also a fundamental tenet of this book that the youth landscape is dynamic and fast-changing. What is relevant this year may be less so next year. Given this research programme was started nearly 10 years ago, some of the material will not have kept pace with more recent developments. It may be helpful to see the ideas in this book as a snapshot of a moment in time rather than a set of 'truths' about young people. In spite of these obvious limits, I hope that people who read this book will treat it as an invitation, and perhaps a starting point, for listening to young people about their own experiences with mental health and mental health support.

Through the process of doing this research and writing this book, I have been very aware of the way that my age, generation and the context in which I grew up, places me a long way from the world of the young people whose experiences I was trying to capture. I have had the good fortune of working on this research alongside a wonderful group of postgraduate students who, for the most part, approximate more closely the age, culture, and experiences of the young people we interviewed. Their doctoral theses and honours dissertations form a large part of the body of research I describe here. While their work is acknowledged throughout the text of the book, I would like to name them individually here in recognition of my appreciation for their contribution. My particular thanks then to Aamina Ali, Emily Adeane, Julia Campbell, Emma Edwards, Rebecca Herald, Yan Yan Lei, Kelly Kerrisk, Karis Knight, Bilal Nasier, Jessica Stubbing, Ting-ya Wang, Jeanne van Wyk and Celine Wills. My understanding and this book have been immeasurably enriched by their data collection, analysis, and the ideas we have discussed together.

I would also like to thank colleagues from the University of Auckland who worked with me on various aspects of the research that I use in this book. They include Claire Cartwright, Jade Le Grice, Fred Seymour and Margaret Wetherell from the School of Psychology; Susanna Trnka from the Department of Anthropology; Jemaima Tiatia-Seath from Te Wānanga o Waipapa, School of Māori Studies and Pacific Studies; Monique Jonas from the School of Population Health; and Jan Wilson from the School of Counselling, Human Services and Social Work all at the University of Auckland. I would also like to thank Pikihuia Pomare from the School of Psychology at Massey University.

This research has been made possible by several funding grants. I am grateful to the Royal Society of New Zealand's *Marsden Fund*, *The Oakley Mental Health Foundation*, *Internet New Zealand* and the University of Auckland, *Science Faculty, Research Development Fund.*

Last and definitely not least, this book could not be written without the many young people who were willing to talk to us so openly about their most personal experiences of distress and suffering, of their good and bad experiences with mental health support, and their hopes for people and services who might support them through the challenges facing their generation.

1 Introduction

Concerns about young people's mental health are ubiquitous in many developed countries with newspaper headlines expressing shock at high youth suicide rates. The popular media are full of stories about the challenges facing youth in contemporary societies ranging from the availability of designer drugs, the pressures of making a living in an increasingly competitive and unforgiving job market, and the effects of social media on their mental health. It is no surprise that young people experience very high rates of mental health problems. Approximately one in five are said to experience mental health problems in any given year, a number not accounting for the many young people who experience ongoing distress which does not meet the threshold for a diagnosis.[1] Despite this, very few turn to formal services for help.[2] This suggests a gap between the support young people *want* to help them with their mental health and the formal services available to them.

As young people outpace adults with their familiarity and use of digital communication, they are exposed to a world of threat and opportunity that is often well beyond the experience of those who are meant to be guiding them into adulthood. Adults concerned with young people's well-being sometimes seem at a loss to know how to reach a generation whose difficulties are very different to those they knew in their youth, and which challenge their 'tried and tested' ideas about how to deal with life.

This situation has left academics and professionals grappling to understand youth and the pressures they face, questioning the state of their own knowledge and practices, and urgently looking for new ways to reach young people in distress. This book explores these issues and suggests changes in the way we need to support young people in today's world. It prioritises the perspective of young people themselves and is largely informed by interviews that we conducted with many young people across New Zealand about their experience of distress and what helps. The aim of the book is to translate young people's own ideas into guidelines for professionals, policymakers, and parents who are searching for better ways to reach young people in distress.

Young people's own views on their mental health provide an important starting point for developing a deeper knowledge of how best to support them. We need to understand their views in the context of contemporary society, the

DOI: 10.4324/9780429322457-1

impact of social and political changes, and the rapid transformations in digital technology that shape the challenges and opportunities faced by this generation. It is also vital to take a good, hard look at traditional conceptualisations of youth mental health and see if it is possible to open up new ways of understanding young people's distress that are a better fit for their own priorities.

Youth in context

In contemporary Western societies, young people are often depicted as 'having it easy' compared to their parents, who worked hard to support their families and grandparents who lived through the austerity of the post-war period. Media reports about millennials (people born roughly between the 1980s and early 2000s) frequently describe this generation in negative terms. At worst, they are lazy and narcissistic, and at best, in need of 'me time' and large doses of praise and affirmation. They are reportedly less civic-minded and more focused on material wealth and success. More favourably, they are acknowledged to be open-minded and more accepting of diversity than previous generations. The boundary between the millennials and the post-millennials — or Gen Z — is fluid, but it is thought that this younger group, influenced by the revolution in digital communication, has shorter concentration spans, is more focused on the present, is more capable of multi-tasking, and has a more global outlook. Like millennials, Gen Z is conscious of the need to make an identity and concerned with success and achievement, although their standards may be less conventional than those of previous generations. This age group reportedly has less respect for formal politics and politicians, but reassuringly they are increasingly showing their commitment to broad social issues such as climate change.

While these kinds of stereotypes of a 'generation' gloss over considerable diversity among youth, they do introduce the idea that young people's values, priorities, and concerns can shift markedly across different times. But for the most part, these popular representations of generational change have tended to place too much emphasis on the internal 'psychology' of generations with less serious consideration of the broader social and economic dynamics that produce changes in young people's priorities. These portrayals also often underestimate the difficulties young people face in their social environments and minimise the legitimacy of the challenges they face.

Beyond these popular representations of generational change, there is a well-grounded body of sociological research which links patterns in youth behaviour and values to changing economic, social, and cultural contexts.[3] Researchers who write about youth from this 'generational' perspective agree that young people face a very different world to the one their parents inherited. Economic and political changes under neoliberalism are partly responsible for this. Post-industrial Western societies have seen less government regulation of the economy and a decrease in the safety nets that were a part of a welfare state. In New Zealand, we have seen a gradual chipping away of the supports that were once in place for young people, whether these be economic, as in free tertiary education or affordable housing, or social and psychological, such as reliable health and social welfare systems. This has led to a greater burden on young people to take care of themselves and a belief that happiness and success are the result of individual effort, a phenomenon known as 'individualism.'[4] In the context of greater economic 'freedom,' there has been a growth in inequality with those who 'make it' often relying on privilege to provide a kick-start for their success. For those unlucky enough to be born with fewer advantages, happiness may be harder to achieve. For example, poverty may contribute to mental health problems in young people. The relationship between mental health problems and economic struggles is a complex one, but Johanna Wyn and her colleagues, for example, show that rising rates of mental health problems for young people in Australia may, in part, be a response to the difficulties in juggling precarious part-time work and fulfilling the expectation to achieve a post-school qualification.[5] Good careers are harder to come by and require higher levels of qualification and longer study than for previous generations. Young people often have to support themselves for extended periods of post-school education, running up large student loan debt in the process. Even with a post-school education under their belt, young people often end up working for years in insecure and low-paid employment.

In recent years, I have heard many stories about young people in New Zealand who find themselves with high levels of student loan debt working for nothing as 'interns' in professions, such as law, that were once considered certain routes to a solid career. Respectable jobs like teaching, which require three to four years of university study, no longer pay enough to support a young single person living in a city like Auckland, let alone allowing them to support a family. Some brave young people go it alone, but the success stories here obscure the difficulty of these independent 'start ups' that often leave young people worrying about whether they are able to pay their rent. Those less brave or lucky end up working on zero-hour contracts in which they must do the unpredictable hours offered with no guarantee that they can cover their weekly expenses.

Some young people find themselves forced to rely on state benefits, often in a context where this is highly stigmatised. Some will leave low-paying jobs or escape unemployment by returning to university for postgraduate studies they hope will open more doors for them. This may work for some, but others find themselves trapped in a cycle of increasing student loan debt and still no career certainty. Of course, there are many examples of young people who have thrived in spite of these difficulties. Nonetheless, it is important to grasp that the world is not necessarily easy for young people today.

Financial pressures are significant in themselves but also lead to other frustrations. Young people are less able to cover rent and, in spite of the almost mythical status given to owning a house in New Zealand, most young people see homeownership as something they are unlikely to achieve in their lifetime. Researchers have recognised the phenomenon of an extended youth in which young people, still studying or unable to earn a living wage, find themselves staying with parents at an age where their parents' generation might have been able to live independently.[6] There are benefits to these kinds of living arrangements, and some cultures prefer this, but for many young people, it is at odds with the rhetoric surrounding the importance of independence. These circumstances can also get in the way of other priorities for young people, such as developing intimate relationships. These arrangements also present parents with challenges, and I have often listened to the frustrations my middle-aged friends express when their young adult children return to live at home, yet again, interrupting their expectations of being 'child-free.'

Besides the direct impact of financial pressures there are more subtle, but no less destructive, impacts from the mismatch between the realities of many young people's lives and their ideas about what these should be. Young people today are supplied with a continuous stream of images which offer glimpses into the lives of those who appear to 'have it all.' This includes 'reality' TV that showcases celebrity lifestyles or media influencers' vlogs on YouTube with their massive cult followings. These glimpses also come from the carefully curated Facebook pages of their 'friends' who post their successes and exotic holiday pictures. More insidiously, in New Zealand and other developed countries, there is a collective fantasy that 'we have it good.' While those who are privileged by the systems they live in may feel that these lifestyles are within their reach, those who struggle with poverty, marginalisation, or other challenges might feel themselves to blame for their own inability to achieve the fulfilled and satisfying futures that seem to be on offer for them. Young people who are just starting out on their own may also be more vulnerable than other age groups to the disappointment and frustration associated with these economic challenges and, even more destructively, the shame that comes from holding themselves responsible for failing.

Sociologists have drawn attention to other broad changes that have affected young people in contemporary developed societies. The economic policies I have just described, together with other social shifts, have increased emphasis on individual responsibility and a lessening of the influence of traditional institutions that governed society in previous decades.[7] The church, for example, has less influence than it used to, governments are seen as bureaucratic necessities rather than leaders, and the nuclear family is no longer the norm. Researchers have described how these changes have helped to break down the roles and organisational frameworks that have given shape to the lives of previous generations.[8] These changes allow greater freedom for young people to choose what they want to believe in or how they want to structure their lives. But while this freedom is exhilarating, it also brings with it considerable uncertainty as the firm (if restrictive) foundations of society appear to be shifting seismically beneath them. In essence, there are more paths for young people to choose from as they build their lives but fewer signposts to guide them. Youth researchers Furlong and Cartmel famously used a transport analogy to compare the experience of previous and current generations of youth.[8] They liken the experience of young people negotiating the process of growing up in previous decades to travelling on a train guided by timetables and tracks. But today, the process could be likened to young people having to drive their own car, with the responsibility to choose the route and to drive safely along it. Essentially, young people must shoulder the burden of building their own lives, taking responsibility for their own choices and facing the consequences when these go wrong.

Climate change is no longer simply sitting threateningly in the background: it is increasingly making its presence felt in people's day-to-day lives. As we go about our daily business we are becoming more aware of the threat to life as we know it on this planet. This is frightening for all of us, but what does this mean for young people with so much future ahead of them? While it becomes increasingly clear that climate change will have unequal effects for those with and without privilege, even in relatively fortunate countries like New Zealand, this is likely to affect everyone. Rob White describes how this phenomenon adds to the general levels of uncertainty for young people and, understandably, righteous anger at the 'boomer' generation that contributed to this situation.[9] Some young people have responded with increasing environmental concern and activism, while others seem to slip into hopeless apathy in the face of a future that seems out of control. It is no coincidence that popular youth culture is saturated with apocalyptic images of zombies and mass annihilation; the zeitgeist captured in the repeated threat in the popular TV series, *Game of Thrones,* that 'winter is coming.'

The COVID-19 pandemic has brought a major threat to the world, resulting in fundamental changes to the way people live their lives, and has clearly shown the illusion that safety depends on a good free-market economy and our own efforts to better ourselves. The pandemic and the lockdown restrictions around it have, in some countries, meant that young people's schooling and vocational choices have been significantly disrupted. At the start of their working lives, with few skills, youth are also most vulnerable to job loss and the possibility of an even more insecure financial future. Through the pandemic, young people have had to deal with their anxiety in relative isolation from their school, college, and university friends. They have also watched the world stumble and fail in dealing with the virus, further undermining their faith in the older generation to know what to do in the face of the overwhelming threats to the planet and its future. While this threat may pass, others will no doubt take its place highlighting for young people the fragility of their future.

I have painted a rather bleak picture of the challenges facing young people and of course, not all features of this new world are negative. There is more openness to diversity in many Western countries than our parents and grandparents experienced. In the past two decades, Auckland, the largest city in New Zealand, has shifted from presenting itself as a relatively homogeneous, white European city to becoming one of the most multi-cultural cities in the world, with increased recognition of Māori as the indigenous first people of Aotearoa and a rapid influx of migrants, largely from various parts of Asia. Young people are more aware of the wide array of alternative lives that can be lived. For some young people, their choice is to identify as 'citizens of the world,' but for others, it is to ally themselves to the particular groups with whom they feel an affinity. For example, young people have a greater opportunity to find and establish connections with others who identify with diverse gender or sexual identities or have similar beliefs such as groups that support animal rights and veganism. Importantly, in the New Zealand context, there is a resurgence of pride in being Māori, and Māori language courses have become increasingly popular. Greater diversity allows many different spaces within which young people can explore their identity and link to others with common values. But while this potentially provides greater freedom for young people, the task of finding a group to belong to may be more difficult than it was for previous generations. Young people today have the possibility to explore or express a greater variety of identities but must also work harder to find these and then to maintain their position within the groups that give them a sense of belonging.

In addition to these challenges, the apparent openness in our developed societies is unevenly spread and sometimes masks both overt and subtle forms of discrimination. For example, gender power differentials continue to constrain young women, with this graphically captured in the high rates of gender violence in New Zealand. This is also evident in the vitriol directed towards young women when they label themselves as feminists or young men when they display sensitivities which are seen as unmasculine. It may be easier for young people to explore their sexuality, but the word 'gay' is still used as slang to describe something unpleasant and many young people struggle to come out with their parents and family members who have conservative views that have not kept up with the changes in society.

The extent of systemic racism across the world has been highlighted in protests that go under the banner of Black Lives Matter. Māori and Pacific Islanders still suffer discrimination on a daily basis in New Zealand and fight negative representations of their people and culture. Migrants, especially those from China and India, are also often subject to overt racism in New Zealand. I have often heard people openly criticise their English, driving skills, or eating habits. There are countless stories of migrants who have not been able to get even low-paying jobs because their applications are rejected on the basis of their foreign names alone. The horror of right-wing hatred towards Muslims in New Zealand was graphically shown in the terrorist attack on two mosques in Christchurch in 2019, leading to the death of 51 people. Across Europe and the United States, there is a similarly disturbing upsurge of populism, right-wing politics, and xenophobia.

In this context, it is unsurprising that young people from minority or marginalised groups are often bullied, excluded, and made to feel 'less than' their peers. In some cases, the rejection is overt, and we hear often, for example, of young people who have been subjected to racial taunting as they walk down the road. But sometimes discrimination can be more insidious and difficult to confront when it is denied, minimised, or presented as a joke.

The revolution in digital technology has also had a considerable impact on young people's lives in contemporary societies, and arguably is one of the few influences which also has a significant effect on less developed countries too. The ease with which people can access information at the click of a mouse (or tap of a screen) and communicate with diverse networks of people unconstrained by geography has transformed expectations and assumptions about social behaviour. Young people can access social networks that go well beyond their neighbourhoods and schools and well beyond their parents' knowledge. Digital communication not only allows young people to find friendship and support outside of their geographical community but also potentially exposes them to some of the worst kinds of homophobia, misogyny, and racism which flourish in the anonymity of online spaces.

For young people who have never known anything different these influences may not be obvious, but they still have a profound impact on the way youth engage with the world. Their expertise with digital technology puts them in a unique position in relation to older generations: a situation in which the usual hierarchies between old and young are turned on their head. Adults are not always able to understand the online environments which young people inhabit, much less regulate these. As youth lead the charge in this new terrain, the medium also changes their views and expectations in ways older generations may only just be beginning to grasp.

The concept of a 'generation gap' has long been with us. Older generations are known to struggle to understand or accept the priorities of the young, and the younger generations lose faith in the ideas and practices of the old. However, the rapid transformations in the ways young people experience their lives in recent decades risk widening this gap to a chasm. Unless adults, including mental health professionals and parents, are willing to take young people and their priorities seriously, there is a danger that we will not be able to help our young people with the significant problems they face.

Talking about young people

There are a range of different words that people use to delineate youth. Traditional developmental theories tend to talk about adolescents as those within the age range of 13–19 years. More colloquially people refer to teenagers in the same age group. While traditional literature on this period of development contains some important ideas, this body of writing has tended to focus less on the way different social and cultural contexts profoundly shape the way that development occurs. The concept of youth provides some freedom from the constraints of a narrow developmental perspective and also recognises that the period of being young has been extended beyond the teenage years in Western, industrialised societies.[10] Partly in response to this, international organisations define youth as being between the ages of 15 and 24 years old, which approximates the way I use this concept through this book.[11]

Discussions about helping youth with their problems can perpetuate some unhelpful stereotypes about what it means to be young. Sometimes young people are portrayed as risky, out of control, and potentially dangerous. Public debates in New Zealand, for example, have focused on whether young people who have committed a crime require correction through 'boot camps' which teach them the value of discipline. Media reports highlight 'boy racers' who take chances on their lives and those of others. These kinds of representations gain traction from research which tells us that young people do not have fully developed frontal lobes until the age of 25.[12] In other conversations, young people are portrayed more sympathetically but also problematically, as vulnerable, emotionally unbalanced, and lacking good judgement. This view is conveyed, for example, through concerns for young people as victims of cyberbullying or as unwitting targets for online predators.

Of course, none of these representations of young people is entirely untrue. Indeed, younger teens do need clear boundaries for their behaviour, and they might be more likely to take some kinds of risks than adults — although it is worth noting that the risk of hazardous drinking among New Zealand youth, which receives a great deal of media attention, is at 33%, only marginally higher than the same risks among men more generally (27%).[13] Young people are also at risk of bullying from peers and abuse from adults and may lack the emotional and practical resources to deal with distress. My point here is not that we should be unconcerned about these issues, but it can be problematic if young people are seen as only 'risky' or 'vulnerable.' These one-sided views reinforce the idea that young people must be recipients of adult scrutiny and control and cannot themselves contribute towards solving the difficulties they face.

In the mental health sphere, young people's views have historically been treated with scepticism which comes from the view that they cannot comment usefully on 'what is good for them.' In contrast, my encounters with young people, even those who have struggled with significant mental health issues, have shown young people to be thoughtful, self-reflective, and full of ideas about how youth mental health services can be improved. Throughout this book, I argue that it is not only morally important to include young people in efforts to address their problems but also given the limited access that adults have to the worlds of young people in contemporary society, they are an essential and valuable resource in the development of our knowledge of youth mental health. More pragmatically, if the key objective is to facilitate young people's use of mental health support that works for them, we must engage directly with the way they see the world, their priorities, and concerns.

Paradoxically, while youth are seen as needing care and control, there is an equally unhelpful counterview which positions young people as totally responsible for managing their circumstances and determining their futures. It is not uncommon to read about young people making 'poor choices' or 'bad decisions' as though all aspects of their lives are within their power to change. While it is important to encourage a sense of responsibility among young people, we have to question whether a 15-year-old who truants school after being bullied for being gay or a young woman who turns to alcohol and drugs to manage the trauma of sexual abuse in her family should be held accountable for the effect this has on their future. This way of thinking can lead to young people carrying an unrealistic, and unfair, sense of responsibility for the difficulties they experience through socio-economic, gender, or cultural disadvantage that have a significant influence on the 'choices' they might have available. It is important not to lose sight of society's responsibility to take care of the basics such as economic security, assurance of respect, and the opportunities that young people need to be given in order to thrive.

The tension between acknowledging that young people have valuable knowledge to bring to our understanding of their mental health, and an awareness that many of their difficulties are not within their power to change, is a difficult one to negotiate. The position I adopt in this book is one that highlights the strengths and creativity which young people show in dealing with mental health issues, while also recognising the significant challenges they face in society.

Hearing the views of young people

While it may seem like common sense to place the voices of young people at the centre of a book about their mental health, it is surprising how seldom this is done. Historically, mental health services have been developed with little serious consideration of the ideas of those who are the recipients of 'treatment.' Randomised controlled trials are the gold standard for establishing the efficacy of psychological interventions, and while this method evaluates the symptomatic change in conditions such as depression, it cannot explore participants' views on what aspects of the therapy they preferred or what they took from their experience. In more recent decades, however, there has been greater awareness of the need to examine the clients' satisfaction with mental health intervention which has led to the increasing integration of 'client outcome' measures into normal clinical practice. While this takes us in a positive direction, I am sometimes reminded of the old joke about the narcissist who says, 'Well enough about me — what do *you* think of me?' Client outcome measures *do* ask people what they did or did not appreciate about any particular intervention but the agenda is often set by the professionals and the question is focused on what they did, or did not, do right. There is, however, a rising movement which aims to empower service users and recognises the importance of their broader views in shaping the service they receive. This movement has been largely led by service users themselves who often have to raise their voices loudly to be heard by mental health professionals. But, if it has been a slow struggle for adult service users to have their voices heard in the area of mental health, this has been even more challenging for young people who have traditionally been treated as unreliable informants on their own well-being and support needs.

While providing a space for young service users' experiences with mental health services may help us to develop approaches which are a better fit for their needs, this is still a rather narrow way of thinking about supporting young people in distress. I am using the word mental health to define the focus of this book, but in reality, the issue requires a broader lens. We need to understand how young people experience their world, what they count as distressing, and how they understand this to affect them. There is a useful body of literature, largely developed in medical anthropology, which focuses on how 'lay people' understand mental health problems, recognising that their point of view may be significantly different to professional views.[14] There is, however, little literature, which looks at 'lay' perspectives among young people specifically, and there are questions about the extent to which the language of mental health is a good fit for the way youth perceive and experience their problems. We also know far too little about the sources of young people's distress in contemporary society and the journeys they take in dealing with mental health issues without professional oversight or intervention. This book aims to provide insight into the sorts of things young people experience as distressing and how they conceptualise this distress. It will also explore young people's preferences in relation to professional services, their encounters with these services, as well as alternative strategies they use to manage their own difficulties, both on- and offline.

Talking about youth mental health

Youth has long been depicted as a time of turbulent emotion or 'sturm and drang' as it was first described by G. Stanley Hall in 1904.[15] Although more recent research has challenged the idea that adolescence is always emotionally difficult, there remains a general perception that young people do experience more distress than people in other age groups, a view given support by the fact that mental health problem is common during this period of life and that many ongoing mental health problems first become apparent in this time.[2] In spite of this perception, young people's distress has not always been labelled as a mental health problem.

In earlier decades, emotional distress or problem behaviour was seen as a manifestation of character weakness to be dealt with through discipline. In industrialised Western societies, however, there has been an increasing shift towards a medicalised understanding of young people's difficulties, with the expectation that problems should be dealt with by a health professional. These kinds of changes can be clearly seen in the historical shifts in the representation of suicide: once seen as a sin, then as a crime, and now is most often attributed to mental health problems.[16] The example of suicide shows how this shift removes some of the negative representations of suicide which contributed to the stigma surrounding this in previous generations. Nevertheless, like all improvements, it brings its own challenges.

Understanding distress or suicide as a mental health problem, within the same framework as physical illness, was intended to reduce stigma but ironically some research has shown that it can actually increase it.[17] This medical view of distress can also easily distract us from the very real difficulties that contribute to young people's distress and pathologises what might be 'normal' reactions to these. Perhaps most importantly when thinking about how to engage young people with support, this medical view of distress may not fit very well with young people's own understandings of distress. Terms like 'depression' and 'psychosis' may well be more frightening and alienating for young people than they are helpful.

In thinking about the relevance of professional mental health knowledge for young people, it is also important to be reminded that youth in contemporary societies are no longer reliant on formal knowledge sources such as doctors, psychologists, or counsellors. The internet has given youth access to a wide range of views from different sources including online communities with other young people who are able to share their own experiences about what works or does not work for them. Professionals often have little knowledge about the wealth of information that young people have at their fingertips and how this influences their understanding of mental health and what support they might need.

If we are to be able to reach young people with support, we need to be able to understand and talk their language of distress. This book explores and identifies some of the ways that young people understand distress, including important issues like suicide.

Youth mental health services

As New Zealand, and many other countries, pays increasing attention to youth mental health, there are calls for more resources to be directed towards services for young people. Youth mental health services are generally recognised to be needed to cover a broad spectrum of difficulties. It is important to provide services for young people with serious mental health problems, but there is also growing awareness of the need for services that can provide early intervention for young people to prevent them from developing more serious mental health problems. In addition, young people need support that can help them to deal with the ordinary 'problems of living' which challenge their well-being.

To deal with problems on the more serious end of the mental health spectrum, most countries offer some state-run mental health services for young people. These services have traditionally divided young people into 'adolescents' (in New Zealand, this is young people up to the age of 17 or 18) who would be expected to attend a combined service intended for children and teens, and older youth who would attend an adult service. For young people who do not meet the severity criteria to access state services, there is usually a range of what is sometimes termed 'primary healthcare' services based in local communities, sometimes linked to general practitioners surgeries, to non-governmental organisations, or to educational institutions (e.g. school counselling services). This collection of services tends to provide patchy or inconsistent coverage for the needs of this group of young people. Beyond these kinds of services, many countries rely on private practitioners to meet the needs of young people and their families where they can afford this or have insurance to cover the costs.

There is much that can be said about how youth mental health services need to be extended or better resourced, but even without these considerations, there are questions about how they need to be transformed to match the broader priorities and expectations of young people today. The general structure of mental health services has changed little in past decades. A young person is usually expected to attend a 'session' with a professional, often held onsite at a clinic. There is typically some kind of assessment process, followed by an intervention that may be carried out over a set period of time. Ongoing individual therapy usually occurs in a prescribed hour once a week, although there may be other interventions such as family sessions, or consultation with a school, alongside this. Psychiatry has established dominance in mental health services, and there is still a very strong reliance on medication as an important part of treatment together with or in place of talking therapies.

Young people's poor use of formal mental health support raises questions about the extent to which these services have kept pace with the priorities and concerns of today's youth: How does the idea of regular weekly therapy work for young people whose arrangements for a Saturday night tend to be made, changed, and communicated in the moment? How is professional expertise perceived by youth who have access to so much knowledge online and from the comfort of their bedrooms? How do the interventions fit with the priorities and concerns of this digital generation?

There are many different groups of adults whose work is aimed at supporting young people's mental health. These include professionals such as psychiatrists, clinical psychologists, counsellors, social workers, general practitioners, mental health nurses, and youth workers. Because of the differences in the values and training of these different groups, it is hard to generalise their approaches to youth mental health, but from the perspective of young people, the differences between the professions are perhaps less significant than they are for professionals themselves. For ease of writing, I have tended to use the word 'mental health professional,' although I have sometimes followed the young people themselves in referring to an interaction with a particular professional, usually, a 'counsellor,' which has become a generic word for those who work in this area.

Professionals who work in youth mental health are often drawn there by a deep commitment and concern for the well-being of young people. However, over the years, I have spoken to many of these committed professionals who feel frustrated at their inability to effectively reach young people in distress. Even those who had taken the time to ask young people what they need often found themselves constrained by cumbersome and outdated systems that impede their efforts to do things differently and struggled to have their own voices heard against the power of the tradition and hierarchy in mental health services.

Despite the challenges of changing the ethos of the mental health services, there are some hopeful advances in the field of youth mental health. The International Declaration on Youth Mental Health was launched in 2012, calling for more appropriate services for young people.[18] This declaration, which included input from professionals and from young people themselves, has propelled the development of several prototypes of youth-friendly services in a number of different countries, that better match the needs of young people today. This book is intended to contribute towards this growing movement exploring mental health through the eyes of young people themselves and asking them what support would work for them.

Researching young people's priorities for mental health support

The starting point for this book is a recognition that young people are actively engaged in making sense of their distress and well-being and have strong ideas about the kind of support they want. I will draw on their ideas to identify opportunities to change what we do so that we can support them more effectively.

During the past eight years my colleagues, students, and I have been involved in a research programme called '*The Mirror Project:* Reflecting young people's views on mental health.' The title came from the idea of holding up a mirror to professionals so that they could see how their efforts were being understood by young people. This programme is the collective title for a range of different projects conducted under this banner. Some of these projects have been undertaken together with colleagues who have worked with me on various research studies and others with my postgraduate students, who have sometimes collected the data and analysed this as part of their theses. I have, with their permission, used these data to inform this book. While I take responsibility for the ideas presented here, I use the terms 'us' and 'we' to recognise the central involvement others have had in amassing the data that form the backbone of this book, and their contribution to the arguments I present here.

To date, we have conducted in-depth interviews or focus groups with nearly 400 young people across New Zealand and have collected the views of hundreds of others in anonymous survey data. We have also analysed textual data from online websites and counselling transcripts from services to explore how young clients engage with these services. The interlinked research projects that inform this book have addressed a number of questions relevant to young people's mental health. In our research, we have asked young people what they see as stressful in their lives, how this affects them, and how they cope. We have asked about the formal and informal support they like to use, online and offline, and what they think mental health services should look like. We have also asked for their suggestions about how to deal with big issues like youth suicide and the impact of social media on mental health. The young people we interviewed ranged from 13 to 25, but the majority clustered in the 16- to 21-year age range. We have also, occasionally, explored the insights of some adults who are trying to provide support to young people. Through the book, I use extracts from the data to illustrate some of the key ideas. The words of research participants are presented in the original form in which they were told and transcribed directly from audio recordings. As some of the data were collected through digital interviews, this material is presented in the way it was written in text by young people to maintain the authenticity of this particular form of communication.

Although I have been writing in sweeping generalisations about youth, it is very important to acknowledge that not all youth experiences are the same. There are not only country-specific differences between young people but also important differences among young people who live in New Zealand. Gender, age, sexuality, culture, and class are just some of the broad demographics that lead to differences in young people's experiences or needs for mental health support. This book will try to consider diversity but may be guilty of skewing somewhat towards commonality in young people's experience of mental health problems and engagement with support. The young people we interviewed included New Zealand Europeans, Māori who are the indigenous people of Aotearoa New Zealand, and Pacific Island youth who are a substantial minority in our region. The data also include the ideas of many immigrants from the UK, India, South Africa, and China, among other countries. Most of our participants came from the city of Auckland where the researchers are based, some from other major cities in New Zealand, and a small number from towns and rural areas around the country.

The structure of the book

In the chapters that follow, I set out some of what we have learned about contemporary youth, the challenges facing young people today, and the psychological pressures they experience as a result. I also look at how young people experience and use the mental health services they currently have available to them and the strengths and failures of these. I examine the potential that digital resources hold for supporting young people. In addition, I look at how young people themselves try to manage the stressors they face in their own networks and make suggestions for how professionals might engage with this largely untapped resource.

The second chapter of the book lays out an understanding of the unique stresses facing young people in this generation and traces, in their own words, the impact that this has had on their lives. It explores some of the prominent themes that have emerged from our discussion with young people, including the pressure they feel to succeed, their struggle to find belonging, and the pain of dealing with rejection.

In the third chapter, I explore the various ways that we conceptualise and talk about young people's distress. I look at how professionals do this and how young people themselves talk about these issues, considering the implications of this for opening up channels of communication between young people and adult professionals.

In the fourth chapter, I examine the importance of identity for young people today. I show how making an identity is central to young people's mental health and how challenges to their identity are often the source of psychological problems. I also highlight how attention to identity issues can improve young people's engagement with support and, conversely, how the failure to consider this leaves young people unwilling to seek help from a counsellor. Finally, I discuss how the process of experiencing a mental health problem and the nature of the support or intervention provided can have profound positive or negative impacts on young people's developing identities.

In the fifth chapter, I focus on agency, which is recognised as an important 'developmental' issue for young people. I explore how this concern plays out in the context of contradictory social expectations that position young people as both powerless and responsible. In this chapter, I highlight the way that threats to their agency can be a major obstacle to young people being able to use mental health support and discuss ways that services and professionals can show greater respect for young people's choices.

In the sixth chapter, I describe the priority that young people give to the quality and authenticity of relationships in their lives. I challenge the idea that young people today are somehow less relational than previous generations and show the importance that a sense of connection still has in their lives, and how the absence of this is a significant contributor to mental health problems. I also show the importance of relationships in facilitating help-seeking and engagement with support.

In the seventh chapter, I consider one of the main obstacles to young people's engagement with support: difficulties of access. I describe the features that young people see as important in designing services that are more welcoming to them. I also consider other challenges to access including the processes of referral, the availability of appointments and the geographic barriers to access.

In the eighth chapter, I focus specifically on the risks and potentials of digital technology for supporting young people in distress. I consider the ways that professionals are using digital technology and consider the extent to which they fit with young people's own use of digital technology to support their mental health.

Finally, in the last chapter of the book, I look at the implications of these ideas for the way that we might develop mental health services for young people that are more in tune with their needs and preferences and set out some of the key elements that need to be recognised as part of a youth-informed approach to mental health support. I also review promising developments in youth mental health services around the world. In addition, I explore the implications for the training of mental health professionals and consider some of the challenges that lie ahead in addressing youth mental health.

2 Youth mental health in context: *The world is different now*

Mental health problems do not develop in a vacuum. While these problems may have complex origins in biological vulnerability and early experience, there is little doubt that the contexts in which people live have a profound determining effect on how they feel about themselves, the world, and their future. Young people today face a wide array of challenges that contribute to distress and, sometimes, to the development of mental health problems.

Often when asked to identify the environmental 'causes' of mental health problems, researchers point to measurable socio-economic indicators such as poverty or to life stressors known to provoke mental health distress, including abuse or neglect. But while there is merit in being able to identify these risks for mental health problems at an epidemiological level, this approach does not tell us enough about how young people themselves are experiencing their world and what aspects of their lives they are finding difficult to manage. To reach young people in distress, we need to look at the challenges they face from the *inside*. In addition to looking objectively at the 'causes' of youth mental health problems, it is important to understand the reasons young people give for experiencing distress. To do this, we need to know more about the concerns that young people have for their lives, the sorts of situations they find difficult, and how these make them feel.

Young people's experiences of the world are, however, not only a matter of individual subjectivity. Those experiences which they find distressing are a product of patterns in the material reality of society including economic and political changes as well as advances in digital communication technology. Young people's experiences of distress are also influenced by changing views about how they should behave, think, and feel. These broader social forces contribute to what has been called 'youth culture.'[19] Although the idea that there is a single 'youth culture' has been strongly contested,[20] there may be some value in offering a snapshot of some of the issues that young people might struggle with today while retaining a recognition that there is likely to be more diversity in experience than can be captured here. Our conversations with young people in New Zealand about the particular issues they experienced as distressing highlighted their struggle with the pressure to succeed and their worries about failure, their need

DOI: 10.4324/9780429322457-2

for belonging and the threat of loneliness, and their strong desire for acceptance and fear of rejection.

Pressure to succeed: *We should have our lives sorted out*

There have been considerable changes in our understanding of success over the generations.[21] In previous centuries, success was ascribed to social class: people were born into a certain status and largely remained there. Later, this idea of success or social standing was seen as a product of luck, certainly admired but not to be attained by the majority. However, many of the young people we spoke to seemed to feel that 'being successful' was a requirement for all young people today. When we interviewed high school students in Auckland about what they found difficult in their lives, many emphasised what they saw as continuous pressure to 'do well.' One young person explained how she felt that everyone was expected to stand out from the crowd:

> cause there's so many people that are doing great things and you, like as an individual you want to be noticed. Not noticed in a bad way but you want to at least be complimented on something, acknowledged in something. And then when there's all that pressure of like everyone's great you want to be up there as well so that your work or something that you've done is noticed.[a]

In this environment, there seemed to be little option for young people to just be doing 'okay.' It is no coincidence that the word 'average' is often used in New Zealand as an insult, an acceptance of mediocrity.

Young people spoke about how the pressure to succeed began at school. They described an education system that allowed little space for diversity in young people's academic ability, measuring them publicly against the same relentless standards. This was the subject of considerable discussion in focus groups in which we asked young people about the sorts of pressures that contributed to our high youth suicide rates in New Zealand.[22]

In the 1990s, New Zealand introduced a strong focus on measuring student outcomes and ensuring that these met uniform standards. This resulted in what has been called a 'frenzy of assessment.'[23] For students in New Zealand, their last three years of school are dominated by external examinations and assignments. School systems in countries like Australia and the United Kingdom place similar pressure on young people, and suicides of young people have been noted as a significant risk during examination periods.[24]

Many of the young people we spoke to felt that their parents were the main drivers of the achievement pressure they faced. One of the young men we interviewed captured this in his recounted conversation with a suicidal friend:

> He told me that it was because he was feeling a lot of pressure to achieve big things or to be really good in school to make his parents proud and to just achieve a lot. And if he wasn't able to do that then he didn't want to go on.[b]

While some young European New Zealanders — who might be thought of as relatively privileged — described their own pressures to succeed, the children of migrant families seemed to experience a very particular set of demands. We interviewed Chinese migrants about the stresses they faced in their lives. These high school students explained their sense that they carried the burden of their parents' migration sacrifice and the expectation that they should not only succeed academically but also succeed across all areas of their lives:

> [My parents] always compared me to my dad's friend's son who was incredibly smart. He always gets 90% in all his sciences and stuff. He plays piano and in year seven he was already like grade six or something. He played a bit of violin. And he did chess and was pretty good at that.[c]

Young Pacific Islanders whose parents had migrated to New Zealand, and were often forced into low paid employment, faced similar demands:

> So, like the way my Samoan family fully works, 100%, is like every generation has to be better than the one that raised them.... It's not about what I want to do now. It's about what's going to make you more successful than they were.[a]

In managing the academic demands of school, young people seemed to have a clear eye on the future, often giving the sense that a failure at school would have an irreversible impact on their adult lives:

> Yeah, it's just that the stress of life, like everyone goes, "Crap I have to do well at school so I can get an 'A,' go to university, get a good job that pays enough money which means I can live comfortably. Nobody wants, yeah, "I'll do crap at everything and live on the streets for the rest of my life." Everybody feels sort of, that social pressure to do well.[a]

This example may sound like an over-estimation of the negative consequences that might flow from a lack of success at school, but I have frequently heard this sentiment mirrored in the concerns of parents who talk with me about their high school-aged children: 'If he drops maths now he will never be able to get a good job.' 'She needs a top grade so she can get into medicine.' This idea that any mistakes you make at school will follow you through your life places a tremendous burden on young people to meet expectations. The way that relatively minor decisions about what subject to take through to the end of school become fraught with anxiety is clearly captured in this extract from one young woman's description of a time she had felt suicidal:

> I tried to harm myself when I was in high school because like it was so stressful and I had to make huge decisions like would I choose science or

> choose arts. That was a huge decision for me at that time. And then I just like, because I like science but I hate physics and I have to do physics. So it's like I don't know what to do. But at that time there is five subjects I have to tell the teacher that I want to do.[b]

Although relatively few young people will occupy the privileged echelons of professional employment, this was something that many felt that they should be doing. One young woman described how everyone around her seemed to be excelling, and the pressure she felt in being exposed to this on social media:

> They either study things like law or medicine or engineering and they generally all have really good grades and they do a whole bunch of extracurricular things. But basically they are very like driven people, and they are the kind of people that you look at on social media and you kind of think this person has it all.[b]

While these professional career possibilities seem a reasonable expectation for some privileged groups of young people, as a university teacher I often see the challenges that face even this fortunate group of young people. I have witnessed the disappointment of the student who enters law and does not make it through into that all-important second year, and the young woman who excelled at school hopes to do medicine but finds she cannot cope with chemistry at the university level. Beyond this group of young people, of course, are the many more who do not even make it to the door of university and feel that they fail from the start.

Ironically, while the future is so much less certain for young people today, they describe a paradoxical pressure to have absolute certainty about their lives as one young woman eloquently described:

> We are always being told that we need to think about our futures, without getting much help in regards to actually planning the future … and so we are put into this perpetual loop of stress, and thinking about the unknown…and when combined with our stress about school and feeling of inadequacy, this all builds up, and so we don't want to think about our futures if we feel like we won't be able to make a decent life for ourselves… This stresses many teenagers out. And we feel like as soon as we turn 20 we should have our lives sorted out; we are often not told the truth: that nobody has her life sorted out at 20…[d]

While the current generation appears to value freedom, research indicates that they still prioritise secure employment above all else.[25] The pressure to know what you want to do and to hit the ground running at university seemed to have left these young people with very little room for considering their career options. Instead, they find themselves on a treadmill of achievement, hurtling along towards goals that they did not necessarily want:

> Like say you didn't know what you want to do next year, you want to take a gap year or just a breather or something. But they're like, "You should take this, you can be a nurse, you can be a doctor, you can be this, you can be this." Like yes, I can be all those things, but is that what I want?[a]

In combination, these factors place enormous pressure on young people. The pressure their parents put on them to succeed is internalised and quickly turns into young people's own expectations of themselves as the extract below captures:

> Yeah sometimes it's like because you are growing up in that pressure system, so perhaps like your parents don't give you pressure but you put pressure on yourself. Like you want to be outstanding, you want to do this, you want to do that and you want to be the top student. You just get used to it. Even though nobody tells you, perhaps you just need someone to tell you like: "Oh you have already done a good job. You don't really have to push yourself like that." But kind of just we get used to it. We have to push ourselves.[b]

In fairness, the rhetoric of success in New Zealand recognises that it is possible to achieve in non-academic ways. Sport, in particular, has a special place in this country and, in some parts of our society, success in art and music are also seen as something to aspire to. On the surface, this seems to provide young people with a range of ways that they can demonstrate their talents. But in reality, these things often become yet another way that young people are expected to succeed. I was travelling home from work on the ferry as I usually do when I overheard two men grumbling about how they would have to spend another weekend taking their children to various sporting activities, but as they did they also showed obvious pride in their children's achievements: "She was in the nationals last year, you know," one said casually and his friend responded with similar reflections on his daughter's talents. As we disembarked from the ferry, however, I caught the wistful tail-end of their discussion: "I remember how when we wanted something to do my mother would give us an old milk bottle and we would kick it around the yard," said one of the men. "Yeah — it's a bit different now," the other replied. This conversation stuck in my mind as a graphic representation of our contemporary society's obsession with success. There is little time for young people to stop and think, to make mistakes, to play, or to explore.

While many of the young people we spoke to emphasise their own responsibility for success or failure, this gives a rather misleading view of the relative freedom young people have to achieve their dreams. It was clear that some of the young people we spoke to were carrying heavy family or financial responsibilities alongside their own education. One young woman explained how she struggled to fit in her schoolwork among her other commitments:

> I was helping out with all the bills, paying the water bill and everything. And you know, any extra shifts that I could, I would take it even if it was like an after school one. So it was, it was tiring spending a whole day at school and then working till like 9 o'clock nd then coming home, sleeping and then doing the whole thing the next day.[a]

While most of those we spoke to focused on the importance of being successful, failure was the ever-present spectre behind this. We did not hear much overt discussion about failure and it may be that the sort of young people who volunteer to talk to researchers have more hope and expectation than those whose voices we do not often hear. These would be the many young people in our society who have given up on success, incapacitated by mental health problems, perhaps living on the streets, or being seen in the youth justice system. These are the casualties of a set of values that not only traps some young people in a pressure cooker of expectation but also relegates those who cannot achieve to the scrapheap.

Looking for belonging: *When I feel isolated that is the worst*

Johanna Wyn and her colleagues have drawn attention to the importance a sense of belonging has in the lives of young people.[26] Their research shows how young people actively seek out relationships and places that they can connect to; attachments that counter the individualising thrust of contemporary society and which help them to manage the, often difficult, transition into adulthood. But there can be challenges for young people in finding a sense of belonging in today's world. In previous generations, belonging was automatically offered to people by virtue of the institutions through which they lived their lives. For the most part, our grandparents did not have to actively *try* to belong, they simply *did* belong, perhaps to a family, to a church, to a village, or even to the company where many spent their whole working lives. Today's youth, on the other hand, have to actively seek out groups, institutions, or places where they can feel they fit.

During adolescence, at least in Western culture, the family is expected to decrease in priority and friends take on more significance as young people turn to their same-age peers for a sense of belonging.[27] We were not surprised then to find in our conversations with young people that friendship provided the foundation for much of their lives. Our interviews with young people were littered with references to friends and friend groups, to the activities and interests they shared, the discussions they had, and the support they gave one another.

While there is a tendency to portray the young people of today as less socially connected than previous generations (and more attached to their phones), for the young people we spoke to, connections to friends were represented as fundamental to their lives and happiness. The young people we interviewed seemed to be searching for genuine connection and aware that 'popularity' did not necessarily equate to this. In our discussions on suicide, there were many examples in which young people seemed to recognise that the appearance of 'having a lot of friends' could still leave them feeling very much alone. As one young man put it:

> And it could be that they have tons of friends but I think there is a different type … it's a different type of loneliness than like lack of social interaction.[b]

He, along with others, clearly recognised the value of having genuine friends, who were loyal and who really cared about them, whether they were talking intensely with them about things that mattered in their lives or just 'hanging out.'

Given the significance of friendship in the lives of young people, it is hardly surprising that some of their most distressing experiences arise in response to difficulties in friendships or, worse, the absence of friends. Many of the young people who have come to see me in therapy over the years have come in the aftermath of falling out with a friendship group, something that seems to occur particularly often among girl friendship groups. I recall one young woman telling me how she had been ostracised by her friends after she had been seen to be talking to one of their boyfriends. She was not even aware of her apparent misdemeanour but arrived to sit with her normal lunch group only to find no one had left a seat for her and not one of her previous 'friends' would look at her. She sat alone at lunch for months, telling no one of her ordeals until she eventually refused to attend school, at which point she was brought to see me by her worried parents. In this example and many others, a transgression of the very strict standards of loyalty seems to be one of the primary causes of ruptures in friendships.

Because of the importance of friends in young people's lives, difficulties in this area have a significant impact on young people. I often find myself explaining to parents who say glibly that their son or daughter just needs to find another nice group of friends and that this would be equivalent to telling an adult that they could easily find another partner when their marriage fails.

Friendships tend to impact every part of young people's lives and even the smaller ups and downs within these relationships can feel overwhelming as one of the young people we spoke to put it:

> If I have had a fight with a friend or a disagreement or I am feeling like maybe they are annoyed at me or something and I am like "shit what have I done?" And that is like anxiety and I have that quite a bit.[b]

Some of the most poignant comments came from young people who had experienced or were experiencing a period in which they had no friends. While some young people end up temporarily in this situation after a fallout with their friends, for others the problems can be a more chronic result of their shyness, bullying, or other reasons. In discussions with young Chinese migrants, some spoke about the loneliness they felt when they first came to New Zealand and how their inability to speak fluent English interfered with their being able to make friends as one school student described:

> It felt like I couldn't make friends with people. I felt lonely, like there was no one else to speak to me or understand my problems and thinking, and stuff.[c]

This understated comment poignantly captures the additional challenges that some young people might have without the important experience of belonging to a friendship group.

Romantic relationships are also a significant part of development during this period and represent another way to belong in a very special and particular way to someone who loves you.[28] Contemporary Western cultures seem, on the face of it, to be more permissive than previous generations. There appear to be fewer restrictions on the expression of sexuality and more allowance of diversity within this. But although this culture of greater sexual freedom seems to be healthier than the strict expectations that constrained our grandparents' lives, this new environment may pose particular challenges for young people. When we interviewed high school students about the stresses they faced, they spoke about the stress entailed managing a culture of 'one night stands' and 'friends with benefits.'[a] Where there are fewer moral 'rules' to guide young people, they have to take responsibility for negotiating this complex environment and for the choices they make. As one young woman explained:

> So, there's that pressure in teens, it's like, What do I believe in? Do I believe in sex before marriage? Or do I believe in like having sex with with a guy that I've been in a relationship with? Or do I just do it so that I can learn in the future.[a]

This young woman's comment also reveals a more general pattern among young people, a hyperawareness of making 'good decisions' about sexual and relationship options. Young people seem less inclined than their predecessors to simply 'fall in love' and instead are concerned about how their decisions might influence the dynamics of their friendship group, whether it fits with their career plans or whether an unwanted advance may be perceived as inappropriate. Rather than 'meeting someone' at a social event or through friends, young people are choosing to 'swipe right' on online dating services like Tinder to make a more considered choice. Even 'hooking up,' a no-strings sexual encounter, seems to be done as a more conscious decision with a clear statement of intentionality.

As always, there are enormous variations in experience. While some young people are negotiating their way through an environment with few guidelines for sexual behaviour, other young people struggle with the clash between the norms of dominant youth cultures in countries like New Zealand and the beliefs and values of their parents. This applies particularly to second-generation migrants to New Zealand. One of the Chinese migrants that we spoke to offered this lucid description of the clash in cultural norms around sexual relationships for Asian youth in comparison with local New Zealand practices:

> In Western media, the ideas such as having relationships in high school, like having a girlfriend, I think white parents are okay with that and don't really mind if their children have a relationship. And the children are quite open to parents about it. But in Asian culture it's not that way, so the ideas that kids are exposed to, their parents won't accept it. If an Asian kid gets in a relationship they usually wouldn't tell their parents and they would be less open about it because parents think it is a distraction from study.[c]

There are more challenges for young people in the Rainbow Community where decisions about intimate relationships may be compounded by awareness of stigma, fears about 'coming out,' and anxieties about the response to a misguided sexual overture. I still recall having a conversation with my flatmate many years ago when we were students. He had just realised he was gay and was talking about how difficult it was to let other people know and to find out who might also be gay in our small university community. While there are more networks available for LGBTQI youth today, it may still be difficult for a young person in a small community to let people know about their gender or sexuality and to connect to communities where they might find a partner. In this context, it is not surprising that online forums and networks have become a crucial source of support for gender and sexually diverse young people.

Nonetheless, despite these difficulties, young people continue to form relationships. When these break up, this can be a source of terrible distress for a young person, especially when this is part of their earliest forays into the intense emotions of love, hurt, and loss as one young person described the end of a romantic relationship:

> I guess I'm kind of overcoming it still, but I recently, by recently I mean three months ago, broke up with my boyfriend of three years… It was hard. And it wasn't a very healthy relationship so it was hard coming to terms with it. But probably one of the most stressful things I've ever been through in my life so far. And it's hard, it's very hard.[a]

In these early romantic relationships young people sometimes also confront challenging interpersonal situations, jealousy, conflict, and a disturbingly large number of young women and some young men also experience sexual and physical violence from a partner. These experiences of violence, control, and manipulation can be especially difficult to recognise for young people who have few points of comparison and may be more inclined to blame themselves for a partner's anger or abuse.

But although developmental theorists emphasise youth as an important period in which young people move away from their families to establish connections with their peers, research is also clear that families continue to matter a great deal to young people.[29] I was sometimes surprised at how some of the young people we interviewed spoke wistfully of wanting to see their parents more. With busy families in which economic necessity requires both parents to work full time, young people today often have less access to their parents than in previous generations. It is interesting that social policy in New Zealand and similar countries often recognise the importance of parenting in the early years in terms of parental leave or supporting flexible working hours while there is much less awareness that parenting also matters as children grow up to become teenagers and young adults.

The lack of access to a caring family was often cited as a source of difficulty for young people. One young woman, for example, gave us this account of the reason for her friend feeling suicidal:

> I would think with her she just didn't have a proper family that she belonged to and I feel like because she wasn't really close with either parent because her father lived in [another country] and she didn't get along with her mum that just made her even worse because she just didn't have a form of escape.[b]

In some cases, parents were described as being too busy to be interested in their children, but there were also many references among the young people we interviewed to the way that the older generation did not seem to understand or appreciate what they were experiencing. Some felt that adults often dismissed the struggles of young people as irrelevant and minimised their concerns, depicting these as 'a stage' or a function of immaturity or over-sensitivity:

> And like, sometimes your family doesn't even really help if you do tell them. Like, 'cause if I'm stressed or something, my dad's one of these type of people that are: "Like, well, life is just going to get harder. Like you're only at high school." He thinks that it's easy. He doesn't understand, like, how bad it is sometimes, so they're not really that much help.[a]

This suggestion that young people are overly sensitive is echoed in the increasingly popular ideas of Jonathan Haidt who argues that young people have been over-protected by their parents and continue to demand special treatment.[30] While this perspective seems on the surface to have some validity, it overlooks the subtle pressures that young people are facing in their lives. For some young people, whose parents may appear to be more involved in their lives, the purpose may not always be to establish closeness or offer protection but rather to monitor their child's progress towards a successful adulthood.

While the refrain of 'my parents don't understand me' would probably resonate with every previous youth generation, there are some marked challenges posed by the gap between the perspective of today's youth and that of their parents. The impact of the digital revolution has radically shifted the experience of the current generation compared with their parents. Young people today inhabit a world that their parents can hardly imagine: it is a world in which knowledge (often created by young people themselves) is instantly accessible, where virtual and augmented reality changes the way that young people experience things and where endless connections extend into the ether. The young people we spoke to were aware that their parents did not, and perhaps *could not*, properly understand the world they inhabited. This is captured in an extract from one of the focus groups we ran to talk about youth suicide:

> So like with our parents when they were our age there isn't as many things like influencing things, like we obviously have social media, It's huge compared to when they were younger. So there is a lot of things like cyberbullying and everything that is that adds to all of that which they didn't have. So, I guess it's kind of hard for parents to understand what their kids will be going through seeing as though they didn't have that.[b]

Family relationship problems and conflict are also often a significant source of stress for young people.[31] To live in a household where there is a high level of tension or violence and to suffer from relationships that are critical and harmful on a daily basis can be unbearable for anyone, but it is particularly difficult for young people who, in most cases, do not have a choice about where they can live.

Schools and other learning institutions potentially play a role in helping young people to belong to something beyond their families.[32] Large high schools and universities, however, may not easily provide the kind of personal connection that young people need. As a university lecturer, I have often watched undergraduate students gathering for the start of a lecture and have been surprised to observe how little social interaction there is between them. Many sit or stand alone, often anxiously staring at their phones and avoiding eye contact with one another. The disconnection that young people might find in this sort of context would be exacerbated for those who travel away from home to attend university. Of course, for those who do not go to university or into other kinds of tertiary training, the opportunities for finding belonging post-high school may be even fewer.

Loneliness was widely acknowledged among the young people we spoke to as a significant contributor to young people feeling suicidal. During our focus group, discussions participants clearly recognised isolation as one of the worst experiences a young person might have:

> When I feel like alone and just sad … I haven't seen any friends in ages, don't know, my mum's in a bad mood or something like that and that that is when I feel like mentally worst … when I feel isolated that is the worst.[b]

This sentiment was echoed in numerous other comments from these focus groups and frequently offered as a likely reason for why a young person might commit suicide:

> Like not having anyone ... just not having any support system around them or like maybe their parents aren't ones to talk about feelings or they're scared to talk to their parents or they don't have friends.[b]

Not surprisingly, when we analysed young people's posts to a suicide prevention forum on the social media platform, Tumblr, one of the main reasons individuals gave for feeling suicidal was loneliness. There were many posts that reflected this, including the one below:

> I feel so depressed and so suicidal. I'm all alone, I have no one to talk to, I have no friends, my family doesn't care about me ... I feel so alone, it kills me inside. I have absolutely no reason to live.[e]

In the face of loneliness, social media was a saviour for some as one young person explained during the course of our discussion on youth suicide:

> Just when you are by yourself in your room at your worst points that is kind of like social media has to be your friend I guess... so it's literally the last thing I check before I go to bed.[b]

Many of the young people we spoke to told us of the importance of a sense of belonging and most of these saw themselves as holding responsibility for being able to find the relationships that might provide this. Loneliness, however, lurked behind their preoccupation with finding connection and many seemed to believe that a young person who was isolated would have no reason to live.

Fearing rejection: *Most people want to fit in*

Developmental theorists have long recognised that young people are strongly invested in 'fitting in.'[33] Part of fitting in is being seen as 'the same,' while being different risks the threat of being excluded. I remember the pressure I felt as a teenager to wear the same clothes or listen to the same music as my friends and the shame of turning up at a party wearing a dress when everyone was wearing jeans. But young people today face a rather more complex social environment than the one that shaped my generation's experience. There is on the surface, greater tolerance of difference and diversity as young people are encouraged to find and express their uniqueness. Under the surface, however, there are still powerful discourses that position certain ways of being as 'normative' and others as deviant. For example, while diverse sexuality is recognised, heterosexuality is often assumed as the norm,[34] and while disability is tolerated, societies tend to be structured in ways that presuppose ableism.[35]

Even while young people are often overtly railing against these restrictions on who they are allowed to be, they often remain highly invested in being seen as 'normal.' When we spoke to high school students about what they found stressful, one of the key issues was how they came across to others. One young person explained how the early years of high school were often fraught with worries about being the 'weird kid.'

> So if you're a sort of reasonable person you try and follow the rules and fit in and just do what you can to sort of not stand out for a bad reason. Most people try not to stand out for a good reason either. I mean they try and get involved but most people want to fit in and not be noticed.[a]

For the young people we spoke to, fitting in or not, depended on subtle markers that they actively monitored as the example from one young person captures:

> Like I remember when I was Year 9 the cool thing was to carry your drink bottle in your hand. Everyone used to do it, and if someone didn't do it everyone was like you're so uncool.[a]

In spite of the fact that there is an apparent appreciation of people's differences and uniqueness, there are clear parameters within which difference is acceptable. One young woman captured the way she experienced this:

> Everyone's like: 'Be yourself, be individual... Be like who you are. But be exactly like us' It's like "What the hell?"[a]

On a more positive note, some of the young people we spoke to talked of the pressure to be the same as their peers lessening as they grew older. They talked about a gradual process of becoming more confident to be who they were and less concerned with the judgements of others as this student's reflection captures:

> But even with some instances that we had in, like, year 10 and stuff, like that sort of stuff doesn't happen anymore. Everyone's sort of like, I mean that's the age where you're trying to find out who you are as a person. And so everyone sort of does different things and people might see that as strange and they mock you for it. But now that everyone's sort of older and know who they are, people are less, because, well if you're trying something new and someone says that you look stupid, they're like, "Oh maybe I'm not so good at that." Whereas when everyone's found out who they are and someone goes, "Oh I hate you." You're like, "Well good for you, I don't really care'cause this is who I am," sort of thing.[a]

But despite this social pressure decreasing among older youth, it seemed clear in our conversations with young people that the careful negotiation of 'fitting in' was a significant source of stress in their lives. The process of finding acceptance may be especially difficult for young people to appear different to their peers or *feel* different in some way. Some of the young migrants we spoke to seemed acutely aware of not fitting in. In conversation, one young person noted astutely how the differentness of being a 'foreigner' resonated with other anxieties that young people have about not fitting in:

> Because a lot of us are foreigners, it's hard. 'Cause you actually don't know what you are and you don't know where you belong or are accepted. And that adds to the natural teenager, "oh I don't belong, I'm not accepted."[a]

Similar sentiments emerged across all our interviews with young people who were treated as foreigners in New Zealand. I deliberately emphasise *treated* as a foreigner because this is often not the experience young immigrants from the United States, the United Kingdom or other European countries have. Racism tends to be reserved specifically for people who are 'visibly different' from white, European New Zealanders and particularly those whose first language is not English. This was a strong theme in our interviews with young Chinese migrants. One young man told this disturbing story of being bullied by his teacher:

> I had this teacher; she was really racist. She started calling me "yellow boy" and stuff. And I was really bad at English back then so she had this spelling list especially for me, and she wrote my full name on it and told me to memorise my full name. I didn't really like that.[c]

There were similar accounts that came from research which aimed at finding out about the stresses that faced young Muslims in New Zealand. In interviews with key participants from the Muslim community, there were many accounts of racism, some subtle and some overt. We heard heartbreaking stories of young Muslims being harassed in the aftermath of IS terror attacks that had taken place in other parts of the world and young women being afraid to wear a hijab in public.

Although Māori are the first peoples of New Zealand, the history of colonisation, marginalisation, and ongoing subtle forms of racism in this country have also challenged the legitimacy of their identity in European-dominated New Zealand.[36] One of the high school students we interviewed explained how she had felt 'different' when she shifted out of her local community school into a 'mainstream school' where there were few Māori:

> I have moved to a white school where it was just a completely different environment and because like in one of my classes I was the only Māori in the class, so it's like, it could be cultural differences. I don't know if they would understand me because they had been through different… I shouldn't say white, sorry, I mean mainstream. I went to a complete mainstream school and you don't know if they understand you.[b]

There would be similar stories from Australia and Canada where indigenous people have been made to experience a sense of their difference, ironically on the land that was once their own.

Fortunately, not all the stories of 'difference' were as unsettling as these. One young Chinese high school student who took part in our research conveyed their pride in being 'different.'

> It's good, best of both worlds ... And being in New Zealand I think it's quite different, like you have an extra something and not just being the same as everyone else.[c]

Some others we spoke to also told us more hopeful stories of being able to be more open about who they were in comparison to previous generations:

> If you think about sexuality for example. If you like the progression in how it's talked about over the years it's become a way more open thing, especially in the youth generation. And if people can talk about it to their friends and they don't even have to say like I'm gay or anything like that, they just go I might be or can you help me figure it out or that kind of stuff, or they just out and out say it, and it's open to talk about and it makes it so much less of an awful experience for a lot of people. Like it makes it so much easier.[b]

It may be that this diversity is allowed more in a big city like Auckland than in smaller towns where there were more conservative attitudes. Some of our participants recognised this:

> Yeah I think Auckland's so good with the diversity because we're like a really big city so the problems we experience, Auckland experienced with like sexualities and genders and bullying and stuff in schools is different to smaller towns where it's more like conventional and traditional yeah.[b]

Bullying has been acknowledged in many parts of the world as being a significant contributor to young people's unhappiness.[37] Strangely, the young people we spoke to said relatively little about bullying as a significant issue in their networks. Where they did talk about bullying, their comments focused rather more on forms of bullying that were hard to call out such as 'joking around' as shown in the following example taken from one of our interviews with a high school student:

> I found out that my friend he was, when he was here this guy threw an apple at his back. And he cried 'cause it's a hard apple and it bruised apparently and stuff like that. But all his friends was just laughing. The guy that threw the apple, like because he's a guy everyone has that, "Why are you crying? Man up!" you know? It's just an apple. But still, like, you know? They made fun of him, that's what makes him sad. And he left, and stuff.[a]

Among girls, subtle bullying seemed to take the form of gossip or exclusion as another high school student described:

> But from my experiences from being at a girls' school, there hasn't been a friendship group that I have sat with that hasn't gossiped about others and girls seem to always want to talk about other girls.[b]

In the same project, one young interviewee tried to convey the difficulty of identifying bullying that happened in this less obvious way:

> Because bullying is not reported as much as they should be. People don't realise that [they are being bullied]. I didn't know that I was being bullied until I look back to it. It's like, "Hey actually they were bullying me." So maybe, like, and some people think like "Hey it's just a joke." Like a joke to you may not be a joke to someone else.[a]

It is difficult to know whether this particular kind of bullying is something that happens more generally within this generation, but it does seem likely that the increased awareness of bullying and school's adopting a 'zero tolerance' policy may have driven bullying underground, where it can emerge in less obvious but no less harmful forms. These subtle forms of bullying can make it hard for young people to recognise bullying and to ask for help.

There is widespread concern about the potential for digital communication to amplify experiences of bullying.[38] The anonymity or sense of distance offered in online forums are thought to free young people up to express greater hostility and more extreme views. One young person provided this example of a particularly cruel comment they had seen online:

> I saw someone on Instagram who have scar on her face which caused by a car accident when she was a child. She posted her selfie anyway with confidence. However, somebody comment under her selfie said "ugh just so ugly."[g]

However, as with their offline experiences, young people tended to emphasise more subtle put-downs and mockery as a source of distress in their online communication. While bullying is not always overt, the fear of being unacceptable to others and particularly to peers remained a significant concern for young people.

What do young people want?

Young people want the challenges that they face in today's world recognised and taken seriously. While it may look like young people today have it easier than their parents and grandparents did, there are subtle pressures that come from the way that society is structured. Young people feel a continuous pressure to succeed, struggle to find a sense of belonging and to be accepted by others.

Those working with young people can help them to negotiate these challenges by

- Challenging the myth that they have it easy today and acknowledging the unique challenges facing youth.
- Helping them to understand that success is not everything and that it is okay to simply be who they are.
- Facilitating opportunities for them to find belonging.
- Encouraging a culture where young people can feel accepted, and bullying and discrimination is not tolerated.

3 Communicating about mental health: *It's how we talk about it*

One of the major thrusts of approaches designed to improve youth mental health has been to encourage young people to speak out about the things that worry them. But in spite of this being the explicit message, one of the single biggest barriers to ensuring youth get the support they need is that young people often do not let others know when they need help. There are many tragic stories of young people who died by suicide leaving their families and communities questioning how it was they were not aware the young person was struggling and wondering why they did not let them know how they were feeling. Much of the research attention in this area has been devoted to identifying the factors that get in the way of young people approaching a trusted adult or professional for help. These 'barriers' to seeking help, as they are often called, are mostly described as though they are a problem *inside* of young people, but we also need to understand how adult and professional ways of talking about these things might contribute to closing down these conversations too. As a starting point, it is helpful to explore how, and where, young people prefer to talk about distress. Understanding this is the key to finding ways to connect with youth and to designing supports that match their preferences for talking about their difficulties.

Barriers to talking about distress: *You are meant to just be chill about everything*

While, on the one hand, young people are told that they need to open up about their distress and reach out for help when they need it, cultural norms sometimes deliver a rather different message. New Zealand, like many English-speaking countries, has a well-earned reputation for a rather 'matter of fact,' pragmatic approach to life's difficulties.[39] In England, this is sometimes referred to as maintaining a 'stiff upper lip'[40] and, in New Zealand, phrases like 'harden up' or 'take a concrete pill' are common responses to public expressions of vulnerability. New Zealand combines this somewhat dismissive approach to emotion with what is sometimes called a 'number eight wire' approach to life's challenges. The number eight wire was apparently used by the European settlers to fix fences (and everything else) and conveys the capacity of this farming nation to use their

DOI: 10.4324/9780429322457-3

ingenuity to make things work with the few resources they had available.[41] While this is usually given a positive meaning, translating approximately as a 'can do' attitude,' it also sometimes means applying a 'quick fix' approach to complex problems, including emotional difficulties.

The young people we spoke to also saw the expression of emotion as a generational issue as well as a national one. As one young person explained:

> My mum came from a very tough, strict family. So, if you had a problem you just dealt with it, you just get over it, you know. "Swallow a concrete pill" kind of attitude back when Mum was our age. But I could say our generation is a lot softer than what it used to be, and I'm sure there's a lot of people that would agree. It's not a bad thing. I guess, we can't really help it.[a]

Some of these generational differences seemed to be particularly stark for migrant youth whose parents held to the cultural values of their home country while their children were integrated into the more permissive culture of mainstream New Zealand. As one young South African participant explained:

> Because my parents grew up in a very conservative South Africa... But sometimes it's a major problem because I am living in a whole different place, and a whole different time to them.[a]

But there are also restrictions on young people opening up about their distress that go beyond these cultural and generational ones. Barbara Ehrenreich argues in her book *Bright-Sided* that neoliberalism is accompanied and supported by a culture of 'positivity' that maintains the myth that happiness is the normal state and that other emotions are an unfortunate deviation from the norm.[42] Psychology itself has been strongly influenced by this in recent decades with the rise of 'positive psychology' being the most obvious example.[43] Positive psychologists call on people to harness their inner strength as they face challenges and to focus on what is good in their lives. This seems on the surface to be a compelling argument, but it carries hidden demands for young people.

While positive psychologists claim that it is never their intention to minimise the reality of the difficulties that people face, in its popular forms, it can create the impression that challenges can be easily overcome, and it is just a matter of re-focusing on the good things. More insidiously, like many other aspects of neoliberalism, positive psychology places the responsibility for happiness on the individual themselves. The notion of resilience, for example, began with a focus on children who seemed invulnerable in the face of negative experiences and then shifted to factors outside of the individual that protected against adversity.[44] In contemporary depictions, resilience has instead come to mean a quality that a person can and should develop through their own efforts.[45] 'Resilience training' is currently popular in workplaces, schools, and universities. Young people are seen to be particularly in need of activities like mindfulness and self-compassion that help to settle their emotions and allow them to focus on the tasks they are expected to perform as productive members of society.[46] This approach is appealing to authorities who, cynics might say, are looking for ways to manage mental health issues without paying attention to the conditions which produce distress. But young people seem less convinced by this argument. In my work with young people in university contexts, I have observed how, when 'resilience' is presented as the solution to problems affecting well-being, this is met by a collective howl of frustration from students who are struggling with unrealistic demands from their university lecturers, financial pressures, and a range of life stressors that are common in this age group.

Young people are not only being asked to shoulder responsibility for their own well-being but also being asked to embrace the many pressures they face with enthusiasm and grace. Angela McRobbie, for example, writes about the way that the ideal for young women in neoliberal societies demands that they be not only successful but also fulfilled in the pursuit of this success.[47] This demanding ideal leaves little space for young people to show the cost of the struggles they face. Nilima Chowdhury, Margaret Wetherell, and I have written about the way this contributes to young women experiencing depression.[48]

In New Zealand, this culture of positivity combines with a template that expects young people to appear to be relaxed and easy-going. This compounds the pressure on young people to appear untroubled by the demands they face. As one of the high school students we spoke to put it:

> Like you're just meant to be like New Zealanders, we have this whole stereotype ... like we're all just calm, like chilled... Like it's okay to be sad but in New Zealand you're meant to just be chill about everything. You're not meant to worry about things.[a]

These combined pressures leave young people trapped in a set of contradictory demands. On the one hand, they must be driven and successful, taking on new challenges and demands, while on the other hand they must also be fulfilled, happy, and relaxed.

The young people that we interviewed seemed aware of how this cultural milieu restricted their ability to speak about unhappiness and described how this permeated their relationships with those close to them. We heard a number of young people talk about how they struggled to live up to others' expectations that they should be content and successful, as one young person explained to us during our focus group discussions on youth suicide:

> Lots of the things we do these days are to keep others happy and we disregard how we feel to make our parents, our friends happy and know that we're okay because we don't want to be a burden on other people.[b]

This young woman went on to explain how talking about anything other than positive experiences was very difficult in this environment:

> I think for some people saying I am not okay is also a step back because like if everyone wants you to be okay and you are saying I'm actually not, it's almost like adding to the problem, like in their eyes I feel.[b]

Several young people we spoke to described how parents often asked them to 'talk' more about their lives, but they sometimes felt that their parents only wanted to hear that they were fitting in with their expectations. As one young woman put it:

> I feel like even with parents, how they are like "Yeah I want my child to be open to me" but when you talk about something they are like "No. I don't want you to do this."[b]

Unsurprisingly, the internet is one of the areas in which young people feel that they need to also display their happiness. Young people's social media networks are full of carefully curated images of other people's desirable lives, their parties, their clothing, their cocktails on a rooftop bar, or enviable date partners. These images contribute to young people feeling the inadequacy of their own lives, the imperfections of their bodies, and social lives. One young person captured the pressure to project a positive life on social media during our discussions about youth suicide:

> About the Instagram thing, it was about having to seem happy right… we are kind of inherently expected to put on a superficial front that is like: "Yeah I am totally fine guys, my life is great."[b]

With the strong message that the ability to be 'happy' rests only in your own hands, young people experience the double whammy of being both unhappy as well as at fault for not being able to make themselves feel better. One young person captured how they found themselves trapped into portraying happy lives online for fear that they would be judged negatively for their unhappiness:

> And also we've got this real expectation to be happy online and in front of everyone else and if you're not it's not like oh what can we do to help this person, it's what's *wrong* with this person![b]

In addition to the cultural expectations of happiness that silence young people's ability to show their vulnerability there are another set of related pressures which are most often acted out in their own peer networks. When we spoke to our research participants about how they responded when other young people showed distress in social media posts or in real-life communications, the phrase we heard most often was 'attention-seeking.' For example, when participants in our youth suicide focus groups were shown a picture of a young girl who had cut down her arms, their immediate response was that this was a clear sign of 'attention-seeking' or that she must be 'a drama queen.' Awareness of the potential for these kinds of dismissive responses to vulnerability or distress clearly acted as a powerful deterrent to openness among many of the young people we spoke to.

Underlying young people's doubts about whether overt expressions of distress are simply 'attention-seeking' is a pervasive concern for the authenticity of expressions of emotion. Young people have become increasingly aware of the potential for things people say to be either 'fake' or 'real.'[49] This seems to be an understandable response to a world where the potential for 'fake' is everywhere, from politicians to media and corporations. In the face of this, the youth have their antennae on alert to spot anything that might be false, exaggerated, or misleading. It is not surprising that this also plays out in young people's evaluations of other's emotional expressions including distress.

The young people we spoke to seemed to approach every public expression of distress with a degree of scepticism. The more overt expressions of distress were, the more likely they were to be seen as false and to elicit an angry or rejecting response as can be seen in this description of a common reaction to someone who talks openly about feeling suicidal:

> Probably initially people go like oh for goodness sake, not again, or this person is looking for attention again… Or like she's taking it too far this time, like "Oh my God she just needs to stop!"[b]

Young people also explained how seeing expressions of distress and suicidality repeatedly on social media seemed to inure them to the impact. As one participant in the suicide focus groups put it:

> I see a lot of attention-seeking on social media on Instagram stories and choose not to engage with it.[b]

The young people we spoke to also recognised the risks of glamorising or normalising these extreme expressions of distress as one of the high school students we interviewed explained it:

> I just want to say like Tumblr especially, like it glamorises [self-harm] but as well it makes it like, it's like the easy thing to do. Like if you're upset, if you just cut your wrists… And it's like oh, okay and so people do it. And I'm just like it's not helping you… I guess it's 'cause we were impressionable and we see it all the time, and it's like glamorised almost.[a]

In responding to other people's distress on social media, young people felt they needed to constantly evaluate the extent to which expressions of distress on social media were 'true' or not. But at the same time, they also acknowledged struggling with the possibility that expressions of suicidality might be real rather than fake, and it would be hard to tell the difference. The young people who took part in our youth suicide focus groups described how they tried to work out whether or not people were serious when they expressed feeling suicidal. One young woman, for example, articulated the way she had evaluated a social media post expressing suicidality:

> I know that [this person] definitely does self-harm quite a lot and has only started doing that within the last few years and that is like something I had no idea about and I think she has like talked about suicide quite vocally. But the thing is like how do you deal with someone like that because how are you supposed to determine whether it's an actual reality for her if it is just a pattern, a trend in her life to kind of just talk about things that.[b]

Another young participant described how she looked to people's past behaviour online to see if they were the sort of person who was normally honest about their lives:

> It also depends on how they portray their life before, like whether they are genuine because yeah there are so many genuine people on Facebook that are like this is my family and this is a not filtered photo and blah, blah, blah. If they are authentic over time I would see one post like that oh well I'll send this person a message.[b]

Yet another young woman who offered a detailed account of the way that a suicide attempt might be understood in two completely different ways depending on the way the person was evaluated more generally:

> I think it depends on the person. Like if someone was really well liked and they were really nice to other people and everyone knows that they are a lovely person and then maybe say if they had a suicide attempt then everyone afterwards would be like they're such a lovely person, don't do that, like talk to me if you need help and it would be like nice positive messages. But if it happened to someone that was say like quite shy and quite introverted and didn't talk to a lot of people or someone who had resting bitch face and was commonly being perceived as someone who wasn't so friendly and the same thing happened to them the reaction might be quite a bit different. It might be like wow this person is so moody or they are just seeking attention.[b]

In spite of being highly aware of the potential for expressions of suicidality and distress to be inauthentic, almost all the young people we spoke to recognised how this attitude added to the reluctance of young people to come forward and ask for help when they needed it. They also acknowledged the irony that while an expression of suicide was regarded as attention-seeking, actually completing suicide led the person's distress to be taken seriously. One insightful young person explained it like this:

> That's a funny kind of situation, like if somebody is talking about it and we're thinking: "Oh well that's just attention-seeking". It's not real and then it's only real when they've done it.[b]

We had a very interesting discussion in one of the focus groups in which the young participants collectively generated an understanding of the paradox that young people found themselves in: If they weren't open about their distress it would be assumed that their problems were not serious enough. But if they did talk openly about feeling distressed, they risked being called attention-seeking. As one of the young men who participated in the group discussion summarised:

> Yeah probably and like the ironic thing is especially if that person is really open about it, like if they are open about "Oh yeah I'm depressed and feeling suicidal" and that kind of stuff then other people respond with "Oh if they are so open about it then they must be attention-seeking". I mean you ask for help but… You're going to come off as if you just want attention… Like in our culture, like "Why don't you ask for help?," and then when you do it's like the attention thing.[b]

In spite of being hyperaware of potentially negative responses to expressions of distress and suicidality, some recognised that this was the only way young people could let others know that they needed help. One young person put it like this:

> That person may need attention, like they may need someone to speak to. Like that could actually be like a cry for help rather than a cry for attention.[b]

Given the pressures on young people that silence their distress, social media is one space where this might be expressed, as one participant put it:

> Or sometimes it's like they are trying to send a message out because they can't talk to anyone, they would rather, it's easier for them to send it out in the media, like social media because I know personally people that do it every day but it's hard for them to talk about it.[b]

Young people's concerns about the authenticity of expressions of distress highlighted the value that they placed on honesty. Throughout our interviews with young people, this seemed to be the benchmark for their communication with others and the hope they had for themselves. While this is an understandable response to a world that holds enormous potential for 'fake,' it can also be a powerful barrier to young people expressing distress, even within the relative safety of their own peer networks.

The challenge of diagnostic language: *You feel like it has to be a huge problem*

Mental health professionals use psychiatric labels to categorise and communicate about different patterns of distress. Mostly these labels are drawn from the major diagnostic systems, the Diagnostic and Statistical Manual (DSM), which is brought out by the American Psychiatric Association,[50] and the manual for the International Classification of Diseases supported by the World Health Organisation.[51] These diagnostic systems are intended to provide an efficient way of communicating about distress between professionals and for linking to research that informs our understanding of prevention and treatment. But while both these diagnostic systems are widely in use, they are also being subject to increasing criticism for the way that they label people and pathologise their problems. The release of the DSM-5 in 2013 was greeted with a particularly strong wave of criticism as people responded to the broadening of certain diagnostic categories as part of an attempt to turn normal human suffering into an 'illness' requiring treatment, usually medication.[52] A recent alternative to this diagnostic system, brought out by the British Psychological Society, The Power, Threat, Meaning framework, is an attempt to redefine mental health problems as a normal response to some of the difficult experiences that people face in their lives but, as a relatively new model, this approach is yet to be widely used.[53]

Some of the strongest voices speaking out against the language of diagnosis have been those of the people who have used mental health services. Service users describe how the labels they receive on their journey through the mental health system make them feel as though they are 'ill' and that there is something inherently 'wrong' with them.[54] Of course, some service users also find comfort in knowing what is the matter with them and that others experience similar problems.[55] Unsurprisingly, young people have similarly mixed feelings about the use of diagnostic language to describe distress.

As a psychologist, I have seldom had a young person come to see me describing themselves as anxious or depressed. Instead, most young people will come to see a counsellor saying that they have fallen out with their friends, that their parents will not allow them the freedom that they would prefer, or that they feel unsure about who they are and what they want in life. This perspective was echoed in our discussions with young people through which they seemed largely to talk about their problems as a normal response to the challenges they face in their lives such as the isolation, rejection, and pressure, which I described in Chapter 2. But while young people tend to see their distress as a product of the difficulties they have to deal with in their lives, they have also been strongly influenced by the use of diagnostic language as a way of describing distress.

One of the recent thrusts of mental health prevention efforts has been to improve young people's 'mental health literacy' by educating them about the signs and symptoms of various mental health problems so that they can easily identify them in themselves and others and seek professional help when appropriate.[56] The point of this strategy is to facilitate young people's ability to recognise the need for professional help. In our conversations with young people, this education seemed to have taken root and their conversations about distress were often peppered with references to 'depression' or 'anxiety.' But while young people used these terms freely, they often seemed to struggle to understand how the idea of distress as an 'illness' could fit alongside their own experiences of distress. A tension between these two explanatory frameworks played out most clearly in our suicide focus groups where, for the most part, the young people seemed to see suicide as something that arose from difficult circumstances:

> I think maybe like when it does happen ... maybe it's because of family problems because he was homosexual so maybe it was his parents or maybe it was social media and peer pressure that caused him to do that.[b]

But from time to time, a young person would talk about suicide arising from 'depression' as the following participant described the suicide of the actor Robin Williams:

> That the brain is low on serotonin and dopamine or like other chemicals that make a person happy, so a person who is depressed is quite low on those levels and a person who is suicidal, it's like dangerously lacking in those chemicals. So I think that it is scientific. It's not purely emotional.[b]

But these kinds of comments often seemed to engender debate about whether suicide was a product of some kind of biologically driven depression or a legitimate response to 'something worse than dying.' One participant captured the confusion that young people seem to feel about these apparently incompatible explanations for suicide:

> You know how you asked why we think people would want to suicide, I think maybe it's not just solely one reason, it might be multi-factorial like maybe they were feeling depressed but they were also feeling neglected and maybe there is just a lot of different reasons that kind of all combined to one and then they do commit suicide. But usually when we go on the news it's usually like depression, drug addiction, but maybe it's something more than that. Maybe there is different other reasons but people don't really talk about all those reasons, so then that is what kind of confuses me.[b]

While mental health professionals would recognise that difficult life events and a mental health diagnosis like depression are not mutually exclusive explanations, for young people these two different paradigms of explanation seem contradictory and add to their difficulty in knowing how they need to describe their distress in order to be listened to.

Researchers have identified that one of the barriers for young people in seeking help is that they worry their problems are not serious enough. In this context, diagnostic language can have a strong appeal for young people. As one participant explained how receiving a diagnosis made her feel:

> It's not just like me making it up, it is actually as bad as I think it is kind of thing.[h]

On the other hand, the idea that it was only if you suffered from a diagnosable mental health problem can leave some young people feeling that they are not deserving of help as one high school student explained:

> I don't have depression or like, you know, you feel like it has to be a huge problem… It's like that, I can deal with it myself, can't really be bothered going up and making a big deal.[a]

Many of the young people we spoke to also seemed frightened of diagnostic language and the thought that it would mean there was 'something wrong' with them. During interviews, young people often talked about the way a mental health diagnosis could make a person feel 'weird' or 'abnormal.' This view was held by many young people but was also seen as particularly problematic in some cultures where mental health problems are seen to be less acceptable or less widely recognised. One of the Chinese high school students we interviewed, for example, talked about how a mental health diagnosis carried a particular stigma in her culture:

> I don't think they [mental health problems] are a really recognised thing in Chinese people, like it's some weird concept … I have a cousin who has depression and my mum talks about it like it's some bizarre disease.[c]

Beyond the formal mental health services, access to the internet has given young people other spaces to explore the value or otherwise of diagnostic labelling. There are multiple online sites that provide information about different diagnostic categories and even give young people the opportunity to diagnose themselves. Indeed, it seemed that many of the young people who spoke about having depression had self-diagnosed. It was not uncommon, for example, to hear a young person say that they had been 'depressed' but had never told anyone about it.

While young people may be drawn to the professional language used to describe mental health problems, this may not necessarily make it easier for them to talk about their distress. Instead, young people might feel that they need to give up their own normalised explanations of distress and take on a potentially stigmatising diagnostic label in order to get the help they need. In other cases, young people may feel that their ordinary experience of distress is not sufficient to warrant receiving help.

Resisting the silence: *We really tried to fight for something to be said*

One of the challenges in creating open channels of communication in which young people can talk to adults and professionals about their distress has been the unwillingness of adults to treat young people as having a legitimate voice in relation to their own mental health. Rather than including young people in conversations about youth mental health, professionals and researchers are much more likely to talk *about* them and their problems in their absence. I have been at many conferences where the discussion has focused on adolescent mental health without any young people being present. One of the reasons why young people might be excluded from conversations about their own well-being is that they are often seen as being unreliable narrators of their own experience and lacking the judgement to know what is best for them.[57] Mental health is also seen to be a sensitive issue with the potential to upset young people. These views combine with the idea that young are volatile and may have 'risky' responses to discourage involving young people' in these discussions.[58] While the intentions behind these kinds of practices may be good, I am reminded of a profound comment made by my blind colleague and friend who had noticed the reluctance of people around him to acknowledge his vision impairment. He explained, "It was as if they were afraid that if they mentioned this, I would suddenly realise that I was unable to see." There seems to be a similar fear surrounding the discussion of mental health issues with young people; it is as if we are afraid that in speaking to them about it, they will suddenly notice that they are experiencing distress.

This set of ideas contributes to invalidating the potential of young people to engage as equals in discussions about their mental health. Nowhere is this issue more clearly expressed than in the way that conversations about youth suicide play out, or perhaps more accurately, are silenced. In New Zealand and many Western countries, one of the main approaches to preventing youth suicide has been to try to control how conversations happen on this subject. In New Zealand, we have until recently had a policy that requires the censorship of suicide from major media and a broad social attitude that warns people of the danger of suicide contagion.[59] Unsurprisingly, in this context many parents and teachers say that they are frightened to talk about suicide. This played out in a scenario at one of the schools where we interviewed young people about youth suicide. We heard how, following the recent suicide of a former pupil, students wanted a public statement from the school's authorities to recognise the distress that they all felt. Instead, they were faced with silence, which no doubt is driven by the policies governing responses to suicide and by the general anxiety around this issue. One young person explained how this left young people struggling alone with their sense of shock and grief:

> There was a cloak of silence over the whole thing and there was zero mention and everybody was completely in shock because we all wanted something. A few of us were really upset about that and we really tried to fight for something to be said, you know.[b]

Their efforts, in this case, were in vain and instead they were given a range of convincing reasons why this could not occur: the family of the young person who had died would be distressed; other students might become distressed; and of course, the possibility that this might ignite much-feared copycat suicides that have been the focus of so much research attention. While the intention behind the decision of the school authorities to remain silent on this issue was no doubt meant to protect young people, it instead made them feel that adults were not willing to talk about an issue that was very important to them.

There is considerable irony in the fact that attempts to control the discussion of suicide by censoring television and newspaper reporting are only likely to affect the extent to which adults lack knowledge about suicide. Young people are much more likely to find out about suicides through informal networks. We were given numerous accounts of how young people had shared information about a suicide on social media, sometimes in the early hours of the morning shortly after the suicide had occurred. For example, one young participant in the suicide focus groups explained how he learned about a friend's suicide online:

> I went home and checked Facebook and there were all these posts about this guy and I was going what's happened and it takes a while to figure it out.[b]

I recall hearing about suicide at my son's school through professional networks some weeks after the event. I asked him whether he knew and he shrugged his shoulders saying he had known for ages. I was saddened by the loss of the possibility to talk with him about it in the moment, to support him with any distress or concern he might have had, or to initiate a useful conversation about youth suicide.

Of course, hearing about suicide online is also not ideal for young people who may hear false information or unsettling details. One young person described how the unpredictable network meant that people did not get clear information in a timely manner:

> Like when I figured it out and shared it to my page I still had people commenting on what I had shared, being like: "What is he talking about, like what is this?" The thing with Facebook, as instantaneous it is to post stuff it still takes a while to trickle through to everybody and I think that makes it more upsetting for people.[b]

Young people also, understandably, misinterpret the reluctance of adults to talk about suicide as a sign of their unwillingness to deal with this issue. We were told by young people that this observation made them less likely to confide in any feelings of suicidality they might have themselves. As one young person in the youth suicide focus groups put it:

> We don't talk about suicide and the conversation isn't open for us to have it. I think that's why we have so many problems.[b]

How information is controlled and managed around the subject of youth suicide is just one example of how young people can be excluded from conversations that involve their own mental health. This situation leaves young people even more dependent on their own peer networks to talk about things that matter to them and less inclined to have open discussions with the adults around them.

Talking with friends: *That's where people would open up the most*

In spite of the various pressures that make young people feel less able to speak out about distress, it was reassuring to hear that many of those we spoke to were actively resisting what they saw as pressure to be silent about issues related to their mental health. Given that adults and professionals were seen to be largely responsible for their reluctance to be open about distress, young people, unsurprisingly, chose to talk to their peer group about the things that bothered or upset them.

The high school students we spoke to, for example, recognised that letting their feelings out in conversations with their friends was a valuable way of managing difficulties:

> Yeah, I have to talk it out and I tell other people you have to talk it out. 'Cause like what's the point of putting on a mask if you're not okay?[a]

In this comment, and those of many of the other young people we spoke to, was the idea that 'talking' in itself was an important way of dealing with distress. For the most part, the kind of talking they preferred was informal, where they could just open up with friends about the things that worried them. One young person gave this description of the way she liked to talk about her troubles with her close friends:

> Like I know like with me and my friends, our therapy sessions would be like when we're just cruising in the car just listening to music and we're just driving and that's not intimidating like we were sitting opposite each other but will get deep with our conversations.[b]

Even when not talking specifically about distress, young people seemed to value the opportunity to talk with others for the sense of release it gave them:

> Talking to people helps, even if it's not specifically sort of about that incident, just talking with someone who you know, who you're friends with

> or you can trust, about anything. Doesn't have to be about that, just talking, just generally relaxing rather than sitting there with everything sort of, like, bottling all up inside you.[a]

While sharing difficulties with a friend can facilitate young people's support seeking it can sometimes also prevent them from looking for help outside of these peer networks.[60] Given that young people turn most often to friends to talk about distress, it will not come as a surprise to learn that one of the main forums in which young people talk with each other about matters related to mental health and distress is social media. There are a number of reasons why social media has become the preferred place for young people to discuss sensitive issues. One of the main reasons is that they can interact freely with other groups of young people without an adult — or particularly parent — involvement and knowledge. Many of the participants in our study looking at support on social media spoke about how they used 'secret' social media accounts to talk about the things that mattered to them. One participant explained the elaborate layers of social media accounts that facilitated private communication in a safe space:

> So, a lot of high schoolers including myself have a "main Instagram account" where they post all their 'good photos' of holidays and outing etc as well as a private second account where we post things we wouldn't post on the 'main.' So i would say the range of number of followers for a private account would be say around 60–120 ish people depending on who you are, consisting of closer friends and essentially people are more open about feelings and showing sides of their life that aren't as amazing as say going overseas, to the beach, party etc. to post on their main account which is open to everyone... i know of many people who even have a third account which would have around 20 followers .... third accounts would obviously be closer friends and i feel that's where people would open up the most.[i]

Importantly, as we were told, these accounts were invisible to the parents of young people and allowed them to communicate without their interference.

Online interactions, where young people often felt more protected by the sense of distance between them and the person they spoke to, seemed to allow a unique opportunity for young people to speak more freely about themselves.

> The main difference is that it's easier to talk about deeply personal things when you're not face-to-face with someone. There's something about that distance that makes it easier to open up.[i]

The word 'venting' was often used to describe the way that young people used social media as an opportunity to say things that they could not say 'in real life' as the following extract from an interview I conducted with one young person about their use of social media suggests:

> I think most times when people want to vent they don't care who's listening it's just typing all of those feelings down and letting it out can be such a huge weight off your chest.[i]

Even face-to-face conversations seemed to be enhanced with digital technology, and it was not uncommon to hear about two young people sitting 'talking' together, texting one another and sharing videos and memes while they sat side by side:

> It's our way of talking. Mostly like all the time we are texting. Yeah even like when we are sitting next to each other, we are kind of just like texting.[j]

The young people we spoke to seemed very conscious of the fact that few adults understood how their communication on social media worked. While of course, many adults are avid users of social media, there still seemed to be some generational divide in the way that this was used to communicate. Older people tend to use social media to post news (personal or public), information about world events or holidays they had enjoyed. In talking with young people about how support worked on social media, young people seem to use it to convey more subtle feeling states, experiences, and perspectives on the world. This generation is fluent in a textual language which includes emojis, symbols, and, of course, the ever-expanding array of acronyms: irl [in real life]; rn [right now]; tbh [to be honest]; and many, many others. One young man conveyed his view that there was a significant generational difference in the way people used digital communication:

> There's definitely a different mentality to speaking to someone online, compared to in person. There's likely a difference in perspective for that between generations just due to exposure to social media.[i]

The language that young people use to communicate about personal issues online is also quite distinctive in its combination of text, videos, and images. One young man we interviewed try to convey the familiarity his generation had with communicating meaningfully using this format:

> The thing though that shouldn't be discounted is the actual different type of vernacular that comes with growing up in the digital age. A full stop at the end of the sentence conveys exactly the mood of the conversation. Even a capital letter, or lack thereof at the beginning of a sentence is telling to the persons emotions.[i]

While young people are communicating about meaningful issues online, the adults around them often tend to view their use of social media as, at best, distracting and, at worst, harmful. The phrase "Put away your phone and talk to someone" might well reinforce young people's fear that adults do not understand this important way of communicating.

Digital communication, and social media, in particular, has allowed young people a space in which they can find their own voice to talk about issues they cannot easily discuss face-to-face, providing greater freedom for them to communicate with each other about mental health-related issues. This is a space which, for the most part, is specifically designed to exclude adults including parents and professionals. The scepticism that adults and professionals often express about young people's use of social media might contribute further to young people's preference for private online communication about the issues that concern them rather than talking to adults.

While professionals bemoan young people's reluctance to reach out for support when they are distressed, there is a range of barriers that prevent this, some of which are the responsibility of the adult world. Obstacles to young people speaking out about the things that worry them include the social pressures that work against disclosing distress, the language professionals use to describe mental health problems, and a lack of appreciation for the ways that young people prefer to talk about these issues.

What do young people want?

Young people want the opportunity to have their voices heard in relation to youth mental health. They want to be able to talk about distress without judgement and to contribute to conversations about how to address the mental health problems they face.

Those working with young people can help them by

- Encouraging them to be open about distress and to resist the social pressures that silence this.
- Using normalised understandings of mental distress rather than diagnostic language.
- Recognising the legitimacy of the various forums and modes of communication that young people prefer, including digital communication.
- Involving them as equals in conversations about youth mental health and suicide.

4 Identity and mental health: *It's who I am*

As psychology textbooks tell us, youth is an important time in which young people make sense of who they are and who they want to be. This development task is often described as making identity.[61] While psychological theories, like those of Erik Erikson,[62] appear to be describing a natural, maturational process which occurs as people move from childhood to adulthood, contemporary theorists recognise that this process is profoundly shaped by the social context in which it occurs. Different cultures, times, and places give different priority to this phase of life and influence the various identities young people can take up.[63]

In industrialised, Western societies, during their youth people typically settle on their gender and sexual preferences, make sense of their values and beliefs, and begin the task of deciding what kind of adult life they want to live. While these kinds of issues have long been recognised as important for young people, engagement with the digital world has given them greater knowledge of the identity options they have open to them and has also honed their awareness of the need to consciously curate an identity both online and offline.

Our conversations with young people often revolved around who they were, how they were different from others, and where they fitted (or did not fit) into different social groups. They spoke about how their identity was sometimes a focus of their distress as well as, at times, being a source of strength in dealing with mental health difficulties. Issues related to identity are particularly important as young people negotiate the process of acknowledging that they have a mental health problem and need professional support. Identity is also fundamental to the way young people understand the purpose of therapy and often defines what they want to get from this.

Making an identity: *It made her feel different*

Young people in the digital age seem to have more options to choose who they want to be. Going well beyond the restricted identities that were thought socially appropriate in previous generations, young people, particularly in Western societies, are aware of the wide variety of identities available to them. Even within the context of family or cultural restrictions, access to the internet allows many young people to explore a wider range of identity options than ever before.

DOI: 10.4324/9780429322457-4

One of the most fundamental ways in which people make their identities are in relation to their gender.[64] These identities may be influenced by biology, but the social environment also shapes the way gender is expressed. Although much has changed in recent decades it seems that young women today still face the demand to be beautiful, and Instagram accounts abound with selfies of young women who are compelled to show themselves and their bodies in ways that emphasise their sexual attractiveness. While much has been made of a 'post-feminist' era in which women seem to have more choice over what their bodies should look like and the kind of clothes that they wear, Nicola Gavey points out how this new freedom is deceptive as young women find themselves subtly colluding with sexist social expectations which hold even more power by virtue of being relatively invisible.[65] This continues to profoundly impact young women's mental health. With size 0 being the desired size for a model, for example, it is a small wonder that eating disorders, such as anorexia nervosa and bulimia, are still common expressions of mental health distress.

Young men also often find themselves constrained by definitions of masculine attractiveness and the relatively new requirement to be 'built.' It is unsurprising in this context that there is a new disorder called muscle dysmorphia and concerns about young men abusing steroids.[66] Despite the appearance of more freedom for young people to be who they want to be, they are well aware of the kinds of bodies that are considered acceptable and those that are not. We can see this clearly in the way that weight continues to carry powerful, negative connotations for young people's identity as this post on a youth online suicide prevention forum illustrates:

> i just want to die. i cant leave my apartment anymore cos im fat and ugly and its summer and everyone talks about how they've lost their winter fat and i have gained so much this past year and always get stared at by people.[e]

But of course, masculine and feminine identity not only is important in telling young people how they should look and dress but also has a strong influence on how and whether they are allowed to experience and express distress. Young women are given the message that they can feel sadness, fear, and anxiety and it is much more acceptable for young women to show their distress openly in tears.[67] While this may seem at one level to be healthy, there is also a double standard that operates here: one in which young women are also often seen as over-emotional and, as a result, their concerns are not taken seriously. Young women, in turn, can underestimate the legitimacy of their own distress and they may approach support with ambivalence, doubtful about their right to be listened to.[68]

For young men, many of the old expectations that they should not cry still hold. Boys more commonly show their distress through aggression, alcohol use, and risky behaviour.[69] This also makes it difficult for them to recognise their distress and less able to ask for help. The idea that there are different expectations about how young men and women should deal with distress came up many times in our discussions with young people about youth suicide:

> Yeah like the stigma that like only women go through this and stuff and like when men feel like this they're like they don't know what to do because it's a woman thing and stuff like that's a feminine thing yeah.[b]

The social constraints that stop boys and young men from expressing their feelings also mean that they often reach points of greater distress before they are able to let someone know how they are feeling as one young woman told us:

> I have a friend, he's a boy and we have a phone call and suddenly he just started crying and it's like: "What's going on?". But I think it's just so stressful but he just suddenly crying. Like because I am a girl we just always talk to each other. So if you suppose like boys and girls they have the same amount of pressure but because girls always talking to their friends, so they just reduce eventually to a balance level. But for boys they just keep all things inside and they just… I don't remember what I said but just suddenly he cried.

It may be that these differences in the way that gender allows people to express distress help to explain the consistent differences in suicidal behaviour and outcomes for young men and women. Young women attempt suicide at higher rates while young men have higher rates of dying by suicide. While there may be many factors that play into this anomaly, some of it may be accounted for by young men's investment in being tough which prevents them from acknowledging distress until the point at which it has already overwhelmed them. One young person who took part in our discussion groups on youth suicide explained the influence of the macho culture in New Zealand on young men:

> Like the Kiwi bloke culture and perhaps it's more stigmatised among males to talk about it than females because stereotypically girls are meant to like talking about their emotions. Girls are meant to be emotional whereas for a guy having emotions and especially having suicidal thoughts or having depression is seen as like an inherent weakness.[b]

The negative effects of social expectations on gender are felt particularly strongly by those who do not conform to the requirement for a binary gender identity.[70] During our research some young people felt able to describe themselves as 'gender fluid' or 'questioning.' While it is helpful that young people have the language to describe these non-binary genders, this glosses over the struggles that young people face in living out these non-normative identities. While these identities are more acceptable in some small circles, there are still challenges in explaining them to others who may not be familiar or accepting of this. Some of the young people we spoke to described the painful complications and challenges of trying to explain who they were to others:

> So I've got all my sexuality friends who are awesome, but with the gender fluidity it's more tricky … But yeah friends-wise I don't expect them to all of a sudden [understand]… I tried a name change with two of them and it didn't work. Same with gender neutral pronouns, I can't expect them to do that just yet.[j]

Diverse gender and sexuality are certainly more acceptable for young people in contemporary Western societies than they were 50 years ago, but this apparent permissiveness again hides some of the real difficulties that young people face 'coming out' and finding networks to which they can safely belong. Many are still in families and communities where this is unacceptable and young people find themselves living inauthentic lives in which they are forced to hide an important aspect of their identity as one young person posted to a suicide prevention forum:

> I can't come out of the closet as gay. If I do I risk losing my family and my entire support system. I risk ruining my life. I don't want to do that. But I also don't want to date guys and live a life of lies. I don't know how much more I can take of this life.[e]

In addition to finding a comfortable gender and sexual identity, young people must also come to terms with other aspects of themselves, such as ethnic and cultural identity. In many countries, different identities come with different degrees of acceptability. Some identities carry historical privilege, like that of white Europeans; while colonised or minority cultural or ethnic identities often carry the baggage of years of discrimination and humiliation. In New Zealand, there is a healthy resurgence of pride in being part of the indigenous culture, Māori, but this is set against the background of a long history of colonisation which has denigrated Māori identity and left many people with inter-generational trauma and shame.[36] As young Māori reclaim their identity, they have to negotiate between the benefits of claiming their own culture and the challenges of a Eurocentric society in which Māori culture and values are often sidelined. This is made more difficult when differences between indigenous cultures and mainstream European culture are often rendered invisible in contemporary societies, and the dominant identities are presented as though they are shared by everyone.

New Zealand, like many Western countries, is becoming increasingly multicultural and many young people identify with more than one ethnicity. These days researchers refer to 'hybrid' identities, which capture the amalgam of ethnic and cultural identities that young people might inhabit.[71] Many young migrants, either first or second generation, are acutely conscious of having to negotiate two different cultural worlds to find an identity that feels comfortable for them. For some, there are major differences of attitude, religion, and practices between their family's home culture and the mainstream youth culture they have to negotiate in New Zealand.

When we interviewed young Chinese migrant school students about the kinds of issues they found stressful, they spoke frequently about the difficulty of managing the tension between what their traditional Chinese families expected of them and the way that their non-Chinese peers appeared to live their lives:

> Europeans are just about the now, just like 'Just have fun, might as well,' kind of the 'You only live once' lifestyle … But in Chinese culture, Chinese tradition, they don't want you to waste your youth. They want you to study hard so then you get a good job, and that's when you can start relaxing.[c]

For the young people who negotiate these different cultures, there are many challenges to making identity as they find themselves pushed and pulled by competing expectations and preferences:

> I am Chinese New Zealander, because we still speak Chinese Mandarin, we eat rice every day, we celebrate Chinese New Year celebrations. But I don't know, I have been living here for 11 years of my life, most of my life, so I quite belong here too … Throughout the years I like eating European foods like burgers, pasta, pizza, although my parents don't like those foods. And also I have learned to play football.[c]

For many of these young people, it is difficult to balance these different identity options. While some struggled to hold on to the advantages of both, some felt that they never quite fitted in with their fellow students at school and instead chose to find their identification with other young people from their home country who shared common values and practices:

> You could say it's harder to relate to white kids because everything they do is different, like their way of life, their mind-set … Whereas with the other Asian kids you already have their mind-set, you don't really have to change or anything, and you automatically feel comfortable being around them.[c]

The decision to seek a comfortable identity with 'their own' can sound like a reasonable 'choice' for a young person but for many, especially those young people whose dress or appearance sets them apart from their European peers, the choice about 'fitting in' is not their own. When we interviewed key informants who worked with Muslim youth in New Zealand, they recounted many incidents in which young Muslims were made to feel different from their peers. For some, there was no alternative but to be defined by the visible signs of their identity. In the context of racism, however, some had sadly made efforts to hide their cultural identity from their peers in order to be accepted:

> Some will stop wearing any outward signs of their religion in certain circumstances. So there was one young girl that would just not wear it [hijab] at university because her friends, it just made her feel different from her friends but she'd put it on on the bus home and she'd wear it at home.[f]

We also heard from a number of young migrants about how, in negotiating these complex identity options, they often ran into difficulties with their families who valued and worked hard to retain their home culture and had expectations that their children would do the same. Many of the young people we spoke to from Pacific Island, Muslim, and Asian backgrounds had found themselves in conflict with their parents and they struggled to manage meeting family expectations and fitting in with their Kiwi peers.

In addition to these 'big' identities, gender, sexuality, ethnicity, culture, and religion, young people also have to negotiate other kinds of 'little' identities defined by what subjects they study at school or university, where they work, whether they play sport, what television shows they watch or music they listen to.

In my youth, young people seemed to be categorised rather simply into nerds who read and attended to their schoolwork, and jocks who excelled on the sports field. This stark division was portrayed in the 1984 movie, *Revenge of the Nerds*, the popularity of which rested on a humorous inversion of the usual power difference between the two groups. The premise of the plot, though, was that you were either a jock or a nerd and could not easily move between the two identities. In my clinical work with young people, I have been struck by the multiple identity options that young people face in today's world, the ephemeral nature of these, and the effort required to maintain them on a daily basis. I have seen some young people, for example, quickly lose their popular identity by not keeping up with the latest clothing brands, not attending the right party or talking too much to 'the wrong people.' Some young people are one day 'in with the cool crowd' and suddenly somehow find themselves on the outside of this, barely knowing what it was they might have done to deserve the exclusion. Identity seems more fluid for young people today than it has been in previous generations.[72] While it is healthy for young people to be able to explore different identity options, the impermanence of contemporary identities also puts a burden of pressure on young people to actively preserve an identity or risk losing it.

In online spaces, identities are highly visible and young people often make the way they want to be seen explicit. They can identify themselves in various ways through their profile pages, their music, television and movie preferences, those they 'follow' on social media, and the kinds of posts they choose to share publicly. In their online lives, young people are also exposed to powerful social media 'influencers' for whom identity is a 'brand'. These influencers work hard to curate an image of themselves which is both unique and alluring. The popularity of their identity can be clearly audited in the number of followers they have.

While most young people will not experience this level of popularity, social media influencers model the importance of consciously shaping online identities. But interestingly, many of the young people we spoke to, especially those who were a little older, expressed scepticism about this kind of affirmation and a concern to limit their engagement with these identity-making strategies. Instead, they spoke about the importance of finding more low-key identities that were more authentic and shared only among those considered to be real friends. But even while this relatively sophisticated group of young people were aware of the pitfalls of this popularity-driven identity-making, they were still conscious of the need to carefully construct their identity. Mostly the young people we spoke to were choosing to make identities which were more private, less 'mainstream' and more 'real,' although perhaps no less consciously curated.

While social media contributes its own pressures to identity formation, it is also a lifeline for some young people who are struggling to find places in which they can express their identity and find acceptance for this. Young people can use online spaces to experiment with different ways of being, different styles of dress, different belief systems, and social networks. Social media makes it relatively easy to perform this kind of identity experimentation, allowing young people to 'try on' and 'try out' different selves, see how they feel, and how others respond. Online communication also makes it possible for young people to find much-needed acceptance for non-mainstream identities. There are many online forums which offer young people an opportunity to simply be themselves in a way they cannot in their offline lives. One young woman, who identified as lesbian, explained how she provided affirmation to another young woman who was struggling to find acceptance for her sexual identity:

> I basically just let her get stuff of her chest because I know she cant tell most people she knows irl about the gay stuff. When I replied I did make sure to say that I care about her a lot.[i]

This kind of online connection has become vital for minority groups who either have restrictions on their ability to meet openly or are isolated or geographically disparate.

While establishing an identity has always been important during adolescence and early adulthood, young people today are increasingly aware of the importance of developing a unique identity, the wide array of options available to them, and the work required to maintain these. The conscious choices young people have to make in relation to their identity echo those they make in other areas of their lives and contribute to the burden of responsibility that young people carry to be their 'best selves.' While digital communication adds to the pressure on young people to carefully curate and develop comfortable and acceptable identities, it also creates spaces to explore identity options and find commonality with others.

Accepting a mental health problem: *I was not the best me*

Acknowledging a mental health problem can have profound consequences in a period in which young people are only just developing a sense of who they are and who they want to become. As they struggle to deal with emotional distress, young people can feel as though they are not living up to their own expectations of themselves and believe that others will think badly of them for not being able to cope better with their lives. Coming to terms with the decision to seek help for distress usually evokes mixed feelings including relief but also often a sense of personal failure. This idea that having a mental health problem represents a moral failure is common to many people but seems to be particularly strong among young people who have been found to struggle with guilt and self-blame when they experience mental health problems.[73] Against the background of individualism, the pressure on young people to self-manage and take responsibility for their own well-being contributes to these negative associations with having a mental health problem. This comes across clearly in a poignant comment taken from one of our interviews with young people who were recovering from a serious mental health problem. This young client captured how she had felt responsible for her own difficulties after she decided to stop taking her medication and became unwell:

> It felt like you let everyone else down and… I got unwell so I felt like I was letting me down because I wasn't the best me.[k]

The context for these individual struggles with having a mental health problem is the stigma surrounding mental health problems in the broader society.[74] Stigma has been recognised as a powerful negative influence on the experience of people with mental health problems and there are numerous campaigns in Western countries designed to reduce this and to present mental illness as 'an illness like any other'.[75] In New Zealand, the *Like Minds, Like Mine* campaign was designed to show people that those with mental health problems are just like them. But in reality, the stigma surrounding mental health remains an issue in New Zealand as it does in other similar countries, even among those who profess to be most open-minded on this issue. One of the most shocking research findings on stigma showed that it is particularly high among people studying in mental health-related areas.[76]

The most insidious effect of stigma is what it does to the identity of people who are its target. When negative social views become a part of people's own sense of themselves this is called 'self-stigma.'[77] For young people who may still be struggling to make an acceptable identity receiving a label which tells them they have a mental illness that can have a negative effect on their developing sense of who they are.[78]

When we spoke with young people about mental health, many seemed acutely aware that having mental health problems carried the potential for considerable stigma. In our focus groups on suicide, participants often spoke about how young people were reluctant to ask for help because of concerns that they would be seen as 'psycho,' 'weird,' or 'crazy' as one young person explained:

> Things like that stops a lot of people cause they don't wanna suddenly be put in this like crazy box and have everyone be like, "Oh my god".[b]

A diagnosis, particularly a diagnosis of a serious mental health problem, can burden a young person's identity with the negative associations of these labels.

This was particularly evident in our research with young people who had been labelled as having a psychotic illness:

> When I was diagnosed with schizophrenia, it was a bit shocking at first. Because I thought schizophrenics were a bit crazy, and I thought, I don't think it anymore, but when you think of a schizophrenic you think of a really unwell person that is senile.[l]

Given the strong investment young people have in being 'normal,' receiving a diagnosis can feel, for a young person, as though they have been catapulted into an identity in which they feel profoundly different from their peers:

> When you are going through an experience defined by a word or defined by a [diagnosis] like bipolar. It's easy to feel like "I don't know anyone else with bipolar, it's just me".[k]

But while stigma can be a significant challenge to a young person's identity, it is important to remember that receiving a diagnosis can have both positive as well as negative effects on a young person's developing identity. For some young people, getting a diagnosis can give a sense of legitimacy. This positive aspect of diagnosis has been well-recognised by researchers who are interested in people's journeys through mental health difficulties. Researchers like Michelle LaFrance, for example, explored the experiences of women with depression.[68] She described how, for these women, a diagnosis can result in an initial feeling of relief and validation. Similarly, some of the young people we spoke to said a diagnosis had helped them feel that they should be taken seriously and that their problems were real. Being taken seriously is particularly important for young people whose difficulties can sometimes be dismissed as an expression of the general turbulence of adolescence. One young woman, for example, described how she felt her distress was not fully appreciated by her doctor until she was given a diagnosis:

> She just thought, I was a teenager at that time, it was just teenage thoughts and emotions and there's nothing really to it, so she kind of downplayed it, which didn't leave me in a good position because it's just like: "Wow, if it's just nothing then why am I feeling this way and why am I feeling so hopeless?".[h]

Taking on the identity of having 'depression' or 'anxiety' can be very appealing for young people and in our research, a proportion of those who had made use of mental health services talked about how they had initially found receiving a diagnosis comforting and had managed to find a positive identity, as well as a sense of belonging through it. But for most of these, the initial appeal wore off as time passed and they were left feeling burdened by an identity that began to feel like a constraint. Being stuck with a diagnosis can ultimately leave people feeling less empowered and less hopeful as they find themselves stuck with the label and the expectations that go along with this. One young person explained how she had tried to resist getting too caught up in her diagnosis and tried to focus on the sort of person she wanted to be in the future:

> That whole sense of finding a purpose in what you're doing and moving looking forward instead of just focusing on the symptoms, because when you focus on them … it can make you feel really like you know things aren't progressing and I'll never be better and I'll be like this forever.[l]

Young people also told us that some of their best encounters with a counsellor were those that made them feel that, in spite of their difficulties, they were 'normal':

> Like it's not really cool, actually thinking you're crazy. You need a professional to tell you, "you're not crazy, there's nothing wrong with you, you're normal". Yeah that's what I kind of needed.[m]

Beyond the formal mental health services, access to the internet has given young people spaces to explore how they want to define their identity in all areas, including in relation to their mental health. There are multiple online sites that provide information about various diagnostic categories and give young people the opportunity to diagnose themselves. In these online spaces, young people are able to self-identify as having one problem or another and find others who share similar problems. This experience of finding other young people who share a diagnosis can be very affirming and challenge a sense of being different.[79] While not exclusively the province of young people, this phenomenon was clearly illustrated in the online forums discussing what it meant to have Asperger's syndrome. Rather than being a sign of something wrong, users of these forums reinvented what it meant to be an 'Aspie,' highlighting their strengths and defining themselves positively in opposition to people who were merely 'neurotypical.'[80]

While online resources can be a helpful way of validating young people's distress and encouraging them to seek help, this can also be a double-edged sword when young people start to define their online identity around this diagnosis. In some social media networks set up for young people struggling with aspects of their identity, for example, we were told it has become normalised to claim a mental health diagnosis and the discussion seemed to sometimes encourage these ways of viewing one's self. One high school student, for example, told us how she had noticed the online pressure on young people to find a diagnostic identity for themselves in order to account for their distress:

> Like when there's like Tumblr and stuff and they have like posts about like depression kind of thing, and then like everyone kind of feels like they should be as well … And then they get these "problems" that they didn't think were problems.[a]

Sometimes, these online forums also facilitate an unhealthy glamorisation of some mental health diagnoses or encourage destructive behaviours. This is seen most clearly in the pro-ana websites (pro-anorexia) which have been accused of encouraging people with eating disorders to be proud of their anorexic identity and romanticising starvation.[81]

The other risk with exploring a mental health identity online is the potential for basing this on incomplete or inaccurate information. As groups of young people start to find themselves in sets of diagnostic criteria, these can lead to unnecessary and sometimes harmful self-diagnoses. Googling 'what type of mental health disorder do I have?' results in a large number of quizzes and questionnaires that promise to tell you whether you have anxiety, depression, ADHD (Attention-Deficit/Hyperactivity Disorder), or even a personality disorder. While many of these websites say that they aim to help people get help for unrecognised mental health problems, it is also highly likely that they give some young people the idea that they have a serious mental health problem when this may not be warranted. For some young people, this may give the comfort of a shared identity with others who appear to have the same problem, but this diagnostic identity can also be a burden which affects the way they see themselves and how they are treated by others.

In spite of some young people being drawn to diagnosis, many recognised that these labels carried significant baggage in terms of identity stigma. Most of the young people we spoke to were eager to destigmatise mental health and many believed that using diagnostic language could increase the likelihood of people feeling that they had something wrong with them.

Making a positive identity: *It was okay to be who I am*

Many of the therapies available for mental health are targeted at reducing the symptoms of mental health problems.[82] But in conversations with young people about their experiences with various kinds of mental health interventions, it became clear that good therapy for them was essentially a journey towards finding a positive identity, one that felt worthwhile and acceptable to themselves and others. Conversely, at its worst, young people saw engagement with mental health services as something that could threaten their identity, leave them feeling less capable, and less certain of who they were.

The young people we spoke to seemed far less focused on dealing with symptoms associated with a particular diagnosis and more concerned that the counsellor was interested in them as a 'whole person.' These young people explained how it was important for them that the counsellor 'got' who they were, as one young client who had used a mental health service explained:

> I think that was quite important … how they really wanted to know about you and they wanted to know what you were interested in, what your thoughts were on certain things.[1]

These priorities do not always fit well with those of the clinicians who conduct mental health assessments. There is often pressure on these professionals to quickly establish the nature of a problem and, if appropriate, a diagnosis that helps to direct the next steps they need to take in helping a client. They also have obligations to assess and document any risk issues for the client, which in practice often involves careful questioning about the possibility that the client might want to harm themselves. While these are important issues to attend to, this can sometimes lead, at least in the first several sessions, to a problem focus at the expense of getting to know the person. Young people who had had this experience in early encounters with a mental health professional spoke about how they left these sessions feeling like they had not been recognised or understood. One young client we interviewed described her frustration with a counsellor who had not taken the time to get to find out about her before focusing on her current problems:

> She asked the wrong questions, like she just focused on what's now, not the past which she left out a whole lot of stuff and … yeah they just take notes heaps.[n]

Other young people spoke about being concerned that mental health professionals would see them only as a problem list. This was particularly difficult for those clients who had been referred to a mental health service because of concerns about difficult behaviour. In research interviews with young clients who had undergone a mental health assessment related to a conduct problem, many seemed to see this as just part of a process in which they were being increasingly defined as 'bad,' as one young man explained:

> Oh, there was a lot, they were like talking about my bad side. I just don't like it.[m]

This young man, along with many others, wanted some initial assurance that the counsellor was equally interested in things they had done well and what was important in their lives rather than just asking them about what had gone wrong.

Concerns about being seen as a 'whole person' remained part of many young people's experience of therapy beyond the first sessions. It was clear that the young people we spoke to wanted a counsellor genuinely interested in who they were as a person rather than just focused on helping them with their problems. One young client spoke warmly about a counsellor who had taken the time to find out what she liked to do and what her interests were:

> I felt like she remembered that I liked photography or I liked reading and drawing and things like that. It was really good to feel like that.[l]

For young people, it was also important for them to feel that the intervention was tailored specifically to their identity. Again, this priority is somewhat at odds with some current practices and guidelines for professionals. Recent decades have seen increasing pressure on mental health professionals to use evidence-based approaches in their therapy.[83] In practice, this is about following the recommendations to use particular therapy models to address particular problems, for example, to use a specifically designed cognitive behaviour therapy (CBT) model of social anxiety to treat social anxiety. It is also not uncommon for clinicians to ensure best practice by relying on manuals that take them uniformly through different modules associated with a recommended therapy. In contrast, the young people we spoke to seemed somewhat indignant at the idea that a counsellor should follow some standard approach to helping them, as captured in this rather scathing comment from one young woman who described her counsellor's efforts as follows:

> It was sort of cognitive brain therapy talking. Yeah she sort of had a set sort of standard to go by … I feel like she says that to everyone. I just feel like she uses that technique on everyone and it's sort of like I didn't feel as though it was specific to my situation.[n]

While she mistakenly refers to 'cognitive brain therapy' here, it is easy enough to see that she means CBT which has become one of the most commonly used short-term, and sometimes manualised, approaches to dealing with mental health problems.

In working with adults, it is common for counsellors to justify their approach to therapy by explaining that it is a tried and tested intervention that had been shown to work with others with similar problems. But for young people, the idea that something that felt as deeply personal as therapy could simply be a standard technique that was used with everyone seemed meaningless or even offensive as another young client emphasised:

> It wasn't just for like, you know it wasn't a set thing they sort of worked with anyone, that at they thought they could apply to anyone who came in.[n]

Unsurprisingly then, what young people seemed to prefer was an approach in which the therapy was designed and adapted specifically to suit who they were. One young man explained how he had appreciated a counsellor in a mental health service who had, at least in his mind, adapted her approach to therapy so it was 'personalised' to match his interest in sport:

> It was almost like you get a personalised boot, if you know what I mean, like a football boot. She personalised everything, even if it were an activity or a relaxation exercise that you can do or heaps of people do around New Zealand or the world or whatever, she made it personal to me.[1]

Young people are aware of the importance of designing therapy to match all aspects of their identity, including cultural identity in therapy. Some young people from minority cultures spoke about needing counsellors who were aware of, and in tune with, who they were culturally. For some young people, this translated into a preference to talk to someone of their own culture as this young Māori woman asserted:

> And so I think it's really important to have Māori counsellors, specific counsellors, counsellors from different ethnicities all over so that we can understand the culture:

> My ideal counsellor would be like a Māori, young Māori woman.

These same views were expressed by a number of Pacific Islander clients:

> Oh because he was *pakeha* [New Zealand European], I didn't feel comfortable talking with him. I reckon it would have been better for me to talk to a Pacific Islander or Māori. It would have been more comfortable. It would have been good 'cause they're from your culture. They know more about your culture and yeah, more understanding of the culture and how the culture thinks and all that.[m]

But this wish to see someone of their own culture was by no means universal among the young people who took part in our studies. Some participants struggled to balance the desire for a counsellor from their own culture with a concern that they would put their confidentiality at risk by talking openly to people who were too closely connected to their families and communities.

Nonetheless, young people seem particularly attuned to what sorts of approaches fitted for them and which did not. One young person explained how she had valued the way her counsellor had listened and responded to her requests for an approach that better fitted with who she was:

> Some of the things that they offered for me to do I didn't really feel were best suited to me, but then I would just tell them that and they would find something else to do.[l]

Young people do not only consider identity to define the kind of therapy that works for them but also firmly believe it underlies what they would like to get out of it. Many of the more enthusiastic accounts of therapy focused on what a young person had learned from therapy about who they were as a person. One young person, for example, spoke about how therapy had helped her to challenge her negative sense of self and how she had come away from this feeling more comfortable with who she was:

> They put things in different ways that made me feel like it was okay to be who I am, but then also it's not really okay. But it wasn't the worst thing in the entire universe. It was just okay being me.[l]

At its best, therapy for young people seemed to be a meaningful and sometimes exciting journey of self-discovery in which young clients came away with a better understanding of who they were and found ways of coping that were particularly suited to them:

> It's very interesting to try to, learning how my brain works and all that kind of stuff. Like if I start to get sad I go "Oh no, I better go do this," like put on some happy music or something.[l]

For some of the young people, counselling was seen as a totally transformative experience which helped them to 'remake' their identities as happier and more confident people who could have the kind of lives they wanted. One young man who had experienced much hardship in his childhood spoke movingly about how counselling had allowed him to move from being lost, aggressive, and homeless to being the person he wanted to be:

> [My] Counselling experience has been good for me, it's changed me to the person I am today. I'm a leader. I play [a sport] as a team captain. I passed last year. I've got my own [car] license.[n]

Sadly, however, we also spoke to young people who felt that their engagement with mental health services had left them feeling not stronger or more comfortable with who they were but more uncertain and sometimes more negative about their identities. We heard about some of these kinds of difficulties from young people who had been given medication such as antidepressants or antipsychotics to treat their mental health problems. While some valued how medication had allowed them to live a more 'normal' life, many still felt that they had also lost some part of their unique identity through the medications. One young woman described how she found herself feeling more muted, less completely herself through the process of using medication:

> What feels different? … feeling like I have lost some of myself and my identity in getting well. Like, I really, I kind of grieve in a way for the person that I was because yeah, she was amazing. I nearly talk about her like she doesn't exist anymore. I know she does…[k]

When we interviewed young women who had been prescribed antidepressants in their teens, we heard of disturbing stories of how those who had been on this medication for a long period experienced profound uncertainty about who they were:

> Over time I just stopped thinking about whether it was the drugs or whether it was me. After six years you've kind of got to give up on that question if it's left unanswered… You're just going to be like, well it's not coming, so I'm going to stop trying…[h]

But most young people, even those whose experience of having a mental health problem or receiving unhelpful treatment for these had damaged them, seemed intent on pursuing the journey to find a worthwhile identity for themselves. While some young people who had had a mental health problem, appreciated the role of professional support in helping them with this journey, many emphasised their own efforts in overcoming the potential for a negative identity and finding a worthwhile sense of themselves. One young woman spoke about how much she had changed since her early struggles, showing clear pride in her new identity as someone who had made it through:

> I was such a mess. Looking back on it I am like, "whoa". A lot of my friends are like "Sarah, how did you do it? What the hell? Who is this Sarah we are meeting now?" Yeah, yeah. So it is kind of like they can see a completely different person. Like, Sarah at 16 and Sarah at 22 are two completely different human beings.[k]

Other young people had also, through their own struggles, been able to find a sense of identity through their own efforts. These young people felt that they had learned to value their difference and could use their own experience to help others as one young person explained:

> I think being diagnosed with something you feel different, but different is never a curse sort of thing you know. I am using it now to get a job and support others who are distressed and change stuff like that. And I really wouldn't be anyone else...[k]

For young people engaging with professional support is a process which has important implications for their identity. In therapy, young people look for counsellors who see them as individuals and adapt their approach to fit around them. They also understand that getting 'better' is not simply about reducing symptoms of distress but part of a process of becoming who they are and who they want to be.

What do young people want?

Young people want to have an opportunity to safely explore who they are and have their identity accepted and affirmed by others. They want the adults around them to give them the space to explore their identity and to actively meet their identity needs.

Those working with young people can help them by

- Recognising the importance of identity and the difficulties young people face in working out who they are and who they want to be.
- Being aware that experiencing mental health distress can be a significant challenge to identity and young people might need help finding a positive identity.
- Responding sensitively to their diverse identity needs during all stages of mental health support and intervention.
- Making identity development a key focus of any mental health intervention.

5 Agency in mental health: *It's my choice*

Through adolescence and beyond, young people become increasingly concerned with being able to exercise their agency.[84] This growing need for independence, often called autonomy, is well-recognised by developmental theorists and, indeed, by parents and other adults who might be familiar with the, sometimes fraught, task of having to re-negotiate 'the rules' with a teenager. As a psychologist, I have often listened to adults who are struggling with the loss of their authority and have also heard young people express frustration that their parents and other adults are not allowing them the freedoms they would like.

While these common struggles are generally portrayed as a predictable challenge for individual families, they also reflect some of the broader dynamics of Western societies. For most of modern history, young people have been subject to the control of adults in the many hierarchical structures through which they live their lives. Schools are a prime example of this. Educational contexts are usually built around the authority of the principal and the teachers, with issues of discipline taking second place only to learning. Young people who attempt to claim their independence often butt up against the rules and, from the school's perspective, a 'troublesome student' is one who will not easily accept adult authority. Even at universities and colleges, students are subject to the power of their lecturers and learning practices situating them firmly at the bottom of the hierarchy in which they must accept the wisdom and judgements of their elders. When young people finally move out of education and into the workplace, they usually still find themselves occupying junior positions in which they have little real authority.

Autonomy and agency are closely related concepts. But while autonomy implies independence from others, agency captures the more important sense in which people feel able to act on their own wishes and intentions.[85] Romantic ideas about agency seem to suggest that this a capacity which develops within an individual, but it is important to recognise that people's agency develops within the limits that society allows.[86] Young people's agency is often constrained both by adults overtly exercising their authority over them and also by ideas that they are not capable of participating effectively in society. Their ability to experience agency is closely linked to the power that society allows young people.

DOI: 10.4324/9780429322457-5

Recent decades seem to have diluted the power of adult authority and challenged some of the traditional restrictions on the freedoms given to young people.[8] Indeed, young people in Western societies do have greater freedom to choose their futures than previous generations, and their access to knowledge gives them greater opportunity to envisage and enact this. But our apparently more open societies also often impose subtle constraints on the freedom of young people. While they are encouraged to make their own choices, young people remain subject to high levels of scrutiny as their success and happiness are tracked carefully through school assessments and adults around them are alert for signs that they may not be conforming to expectations. The popular idea of 'helicopter parenting' seems a particularly apt metaphor for this watchful attitude, which is intended to be protective but can also be interpreted as restrictive.[87]

Young people today are also more likely to experience these more subtle challenges to their agency over a longer period. Given the need for extended education, the difficulty of settling into a career, and the consequent lack of financial independence, young people may find themselves living at home with parents and with constraints on their freedom well into their 20s.[5] Young people today then find themselves in a paradox as their expectations of greater freedom confront both vestiges of the old as well as the, more subtle, new restrictions on them.

If we are to reach young people, we need to understand how their agency and associated power struggles contribute to the mental health challenges they face. We need to be able to recognise the barriers that power imbalances pose for young people's engagement with support and how their desire to exercise their own agency shapes the kind of support they want.

Being powerless: *You get stuck with that*

The emotional struggles that young people face in many cases reflect the lack of power that they have over aspects of their own lives. For example, in families, children and young people have little choice but to tolerate the behaviour and expectations of their elders. While we hope that young people get to live in homes with adults who protect them, provide fair discipline, and allow opportunities for them to express their developing sense of agency, we know that this is definitely not the case for some. Young people can be exposed to all kinds of harmful experiences in their families.[88] Similarly, while school is meant to provide young people with access to knowledge, opportunities for development, and social interaction, for some young people it means being bullied or humiliated on a daily basis.[89] A post on an internet suicide prevention forum graphically captured the experience of one young person who had had little option but to survive a school experience they clearly found intolerable:

> I just want it to end. and to all the people who say "it will end, it has to at some point!" FUCK YOU because I waited 18 fucking years and endless torture to get through high school.[e]

In their homes, young people might be subject to a parent's alcoholic rages, marital violence, sexual abuse, or more subtle forms of psychological cruelty and humiliation. In the same online suicide prevention forum, I referred to earlier, another young person posted about how they had had to put up with years of abuse from their step-father with no option of escape:

> My stepdad does not treat me like a human being like i dont get even the slightest shred of respect or decency from him and ive been both physically and verbally abused by him for seven years and i really want to fucking die.[c]

These types of comment capture the experience of young people trapped, sometimes for years, in circumstances over which they have no control, no freedom to walk away and often nowhere to go even if they did leave. This understated comment from a young person in our suicide focus groups highlights the powerlessness of youth in these situations:

> I know especially if you have difficulties at home, obviously you get stuck with that because you can't exactly leave home when you want.[b]

We see the products of these unbearable circumstances among those young people who find themselves living on the street, where whatever challenges they face seem less awful than returning home. But for many young people, there is no option but to keep living at home or turning up at school, hoping that eventually adulthood will provide the escape from an abusive parent, teacher, or peer. Of course, adults also experience abuse in their homes or workplaces, a phenomenon captured graphically in the high rates of domestic abuse against women, but young people and children's relative powerlessness makes them uniquely vulnerable to these kinds of adverse events, with arguably even fewer independent resources to help them manage these.

Even without these kinds of extremely adverse circumstances, young people still experience a lack of control over basic aspects of their lives, where they go, who they see, and how they spend their time. A lack of power is recognised to be particularly detrimental to people's mental health, and empowerment is often one of the key foci of intervention in projects aimed at improving the mental health of women, minority communities, and other groups who lack power in society.[90] In contrast to adults in this position, young people's lack of access to power is normalised and is treated as a necessary part of this life stage. While some of the limits on young people's behaviour are beneficial and designed to keep them safe, the constraints on their agency may be a source of frustration and create challenges in their everyday lives.

Increasingly young people are asking for greater acknowledgement of their role as active participants in their own lives. Western societies and their structures are becoming more aware of the importance of including youth voices in the planning and implementation of policies, and young people themselves are more aware of their own rights in a whole range of social institutions that affect them, from law to health and education. But while there is clear momentum in the area of youth rights, there is a long way to go before most young people will have real opportunities to exercise their power.[91]

Losing control: *I did not want to go*

The clash between the rhetoric of freedom of choice and the real constraints on young people's ability to exercise this contributes to making them sharply aware of threats to their agency during the process of looking for, and receiving, help. In our conversations with young people, it became clear that one of the main reasons preventing them from seeking help for distress is a concern that it will result in adults taking control of their lives. This fear has some foundation in reality. If young people disclose that they are experiencing distress related to some circumstance, this may immediately mean that they have less choice over how they are able to deal with the situation. For example, if a young person is caught in a difficult relationship, their parents might well intervene to prevent them from seeing the person in question; if they are worried about failing academically, their parents or teachers may demand they stay home and study or shift them from one school to another; if they tell a counsellor they are afraid of their step-father, they may be removed from their home by child protection services. While all of these decisions might be in the young person's 'best interests,' the opportunity for them to find their own way through these difficult circumstances, and in their own time, might well be abruptly taken from them.

It is ironic that these adult interventions which are aimed at protecting young people are also precisely what prevent them from asking for help from adults, sometimes even in very serious situations such as those that threaten their safety. We were concerned to hear stories from some young people that fear of adults becoming involved and taking over decision making was a major deterrent to some to them getting help at times where they may have been at risk of physical harm or other extreme circumstances. One young woman who had used an anonymous text counselling service explained why she had been frightened to ask for help with a violent parent:

> It just feels because I have younger siblings, they might take my brothers and sisters away from me.[j]

Another young person told us how her previous attempts to tell a counsellor about her suicidal feelings had resulted in, what was for her, a frightening loss of control over the situation. Disturbingly she explained how, because of this, she was no longer willing to seek help for ongoing feelings of suicidality:

> You don't know how much to tell and also I guess the consequences that come with it. I have had a few times where they have threatened to call the police for self-harming and suicide. And that doesn't help. It really doesn't. If anything, if um … it makes you withdraw a lot more because all of a

> sudden it's, it gets really scary where it's like oh my gosh, no I can't do that, then everyone will find out, then my parents will find out, and they really scared me that time. And so I don't bring that up anymore. Even if that's something on my mind, I don't bring that up.[j]

In giving these examples, I do not mean to suggest that adults should *not* intervene in circumstances where a young person might be at risk, but I rather wanted to capture how young people's fear about losing agency can get in the way of allowing them to get the support they need, even in extreme states of difficulty and distress. This creates a real ethical and clinical dilemma for clinicians and others working with young people, especially in the adolescent age group, about when and whether to alert parents or other authorities to possible risks facing a young person and risk their disengagement from help as a result.[92] One of the risks which receives significant attention in the mental health arena is suicidality. The guidelines for professionals are clear that they must always respond on the side of caution to ensure the safety of the young person, but the longer-term risk is that that young person, as well their friends who hear about it, might choose not to seek help for suicidal feelings in the future. It is understandable that for young people, the decision to disclose distress to an adult may be a difficult one in which they have to weigh up the relative benefits of receiving help against the threat of potentially losing control over their lives.

Even when young people are able to successfully negotiate the difficult decision to tell an adult about their distress, they might face further challenges to their agency in the decision to see a professional for help. For most adults, the initial decision to seek a counsellor's help is a choice they make themselves. They might take up this option after a recommendation from a general practitioner or with the encouragement of a partner, family member, or friend, but the final decision to make an appointment is usually theirs alone.

There are, of course, some instances in which an adult is 'made' to seek help and these are associated with criminal behaviour or a serious mental health problem which means they are at risk to themselves or others, but these situations are relatively rare. For young people, however, it is often different and, for those particularly in the younger age group, their first encounter with a counsellor or other mental health professional will not have been their choice. Parents, teachers, and other adults are often partly, if not wholly, responsible for making this decision for a young person. For example, one of the young people who had been referred to a child and adolescent mental health service captured a fairly typical pattern in these kinds of referrals:

> Um [the counsellor] asked first but then me and my mum had a talk about it and then she told me that I have to do counselling, so then I just go along with other people. Can't be bothered arguing.[m]

Other young people told us how even when they were not specifically instructed to go to counselling, their 'decision' ended up being a result of pressure from the adults around them. One young Māori client, for example, told us how she had eventually bowed to the collective pressure of adults in her whānau (extended family):

> Um, if I didn't do it mum would like be angry at me, like 'cause she wanted me to do it. Like my aunty, and my aunties and uncles, some of them, like they want me to get help 'cause sometimes I just have those worse feelings you know … Well I just kept telling my mum "I didn't want to go. I don't want to go." [She says] "Get out there, go." [I say]"Okay."[m]

The decision to send a young person for professional help is also quite often tied up with problem behaviour whether it be eating problems, drug use, or deteriorating school work. For many of these young clients, their first encounter with a counsellor or other support worker is closely linked to 'being in trouble.' This is compounded for young people who are familiar with being punished and whose prototype for talking about their problems with an adult authority figure would be being called to the principal's office for a telling off. Given these circumstances, it is a small wonder that some young people can find the prospect of going to see a professional for help with a psychological problem a very daunting one. This was clearly an issue for some of the young participants we interviewed. One young client explained his initial trepidation at having to attend an assessment:

> Oh 'cause I thought [the mental health service] would be like one of those places like, like oh like they would growl at you. Oh no like, people who get like mad at you for the stuff you do.[m]

While some community-based counselling services allow young people to book and attend appointments alone, it is not uncommon for young people to be sent to therapy for the first time together with their parents. While this approach, which draws from family therapy,[93] is appropriately applied in work with young children, it can be problematic when it is used without discussion with adolescents. Many of the young people we spoke to who had used the formal mental health services spoke about having experienced some discomfort in having their parents present for an initial session. One of the young clients explained why having parents in the room for the first session with her had made her feel uncomfortable:

> At first I was, I think I was holding back a bit on information, because I didn't want my parents knowing what I had done. It was a bit awkward, 'cause I don't really like saying like stuff in front of my mum and dad. 'Cause I never tell my problems to my mum and dad.[m]

From a clinician's perspective, there are benefits to having parents and other family members involved in the mental health assessment and therapy of young people. These advantages include being able to understand the situation from multiple perspectives, having an opportunity to observe family dynamics in the room, and engaging the family in supporting the young person to overcome whatever difficulties they have. In my own clinical training, these ideas were central to our understanding of how to work effectively with young people. But having since spoken extensively to young clients I am more aware of the challenges they face in an initial encounter with a mental health professional which includes their parents. Even when adults are trying to be helpful and to make space for their young people to get the help they need, they are unlikely to be as acutely aware of the inequalities of power in these situations as the young client themselves. From the point of view of the young person, the involvement of a parent can get in the way of them being able to talk openly about what they are feeling and constrain their ability to give their own account of their experience. We heard this from a young client whose, no doubt well-meaning, mother had been included in an assessment session:

> I don't mind mum coming, I just don't like her staying with me, because she always butts into my conversations, and then she will like change the story and she doesn't even know.[m]

In some cultures, family or community-based approaches are considered appropriate.[94] Some of our young Māori and Pasifika participants, for example, spoke about how they valued having their family members there to support them. But while this was the case for some of the young Māori and Pasifika youth we spoke to, it clearly was not the preference of others. It was a helpful reminder to us that cultural priorities may not always be held to be equally valuable by all members of a particular culture and that young people may be positioned somewhat differently than their elders in relation to traditional practices and beliefs.

In initial interactions, surrounded by adults, it can be understandably very difficult for a young person to find their own voice to articulate what is happening for them and to say what help they need. This is exacerbated when, as often happens, the clinician ends up addressing their questions to the parents. As one young person observed:

> I didn't like it that they talked about me and looked at my parents. They didn't even look at me and I was right in the room with them … My mum would be there and my dad. They would talk about me to my parents, directly to my parents and ignore me as I sat there. I didn't like that.[l]

The challenges that young people face in actively participating in conversations about their own mental health also come from their difficulty comprehending the language used in these settings. While most mental health professionals are aware of the need to communicate in ways that their clients can understand, they are also steeped in the use of professional language and sometimes lose sight of how this might differ from the ways that non-professionals might describe things, let alone young people. It is unsurprising then that some of the young people we spoke to mentioned that they didn't always properly grasp what was being spoken about and what was being decided for them as one young person put it:

> Just like they were talking in massive words. They were like complicated. 'Cause it's like all business kind of stuff. Yeah, very formal. Yeah just, I don't know, oh yeah they were big words. Yeah that I didn't understand.[m]

On the other hand, young people are also highly attuned to a patronising tone and can easily tell when an adult is 'talking down' to them. One young person offered this astute observation of how counsellors had treated her when she was younger:

> I've noticed a difference from being most recently in the past year compared to being in it when I was 15 … They really treat you differently in the sense that you don't deserve to know what's going on with you and you don't really deserve to know what [they're] thinking about … and I felt like I was being belittled or patronised or disrespected and there's no worse feeling … I've realised they're kind of reinforcing that vulnerability rather than empowering you.[o]

It can be challenging for those who work with young people to find the right level for talking with a client. There is a significant cognitive change between the ages of 13 and 19, for example, but even two 15-year-olds may have a completely different capability with language and ability to articulate their experience. This is especially demanding in the initial meetings in which the mental health professional might have little knowledge of the young client to help them determine the right level of communication.

Specific issues such as parents' involvement or the level of language used during interactions between a young client and a mental health professional make obvious contributions to the imbalance of power between adults and the young person during the process of assessment or counselling. However, young people also spoke about a more diffuse sense of powerlessness as they entered, what for many, was an intimidating situation in which they felt 'dominated' by the double power of adults who were also professionals. One young person captured how she saw this:

> [I wanted] just to have a bit more of a balance in the relationship because it's not really balanced you know. It's too dominant I find. You feel a little bit too controlled and you just feel kind of like what I said before, you're a teenager sitting in a room, with people who've been listening for 20 years or so and yeah seen it all before kind of thing and it's yeah … it's really intimidating.[l]

The loss of control that young people often experience through the process of being referred for help and in the initial assessment sessions is frequently repeated in decisions about their treatment. When we interviewed young women about their experiences of being prescribed antidepressants, they spoke about how difficult it had been to challenge the authoritative opinion of their doctor. As one young woman explained:

> Well the thing with my doctor is she is my family doctor so I've been going since I was little but she's the sort of person, "it's just like you need to do this, so do it."[h]

While antidepressants are known to have a variety of unpleasant side effects,[95] young people find it hard to articulate their concerns and have them taken seriously. One young client who been through the mental health system conveyed the subtle pressures that make it difficult for young people to raise their concerns in the intimidating space of the consulting room:

> She put me on [another medication] and yeah but I didn't really feel like I could talk about how much I hated the side effects because I just kind of felt like I was whining and they would think I was being ungrateful or something.[l]

Young people also struggled to raise concerns about the counselling process or to let the counsellor know what they preferred. One young woman explained how she had been worried that the counsellor was not maintaining confidentiality but did not feel able to raise this with her. As she put it:

> Yeah how do you say to [an adult] "Hey by the way I don't think that's quite right" ... Yeah sometimes you should but I've not got the courage to.[n]

Young people's needs for an agency may be strongly challenged through the process of help-seeking, in their initial encounters with professionals, and also through their lack of involvement in the decisions about what treatments they are given.

Resisting authority: *I refused to say anything*

When young people find themselves excluded from decisions about their own well-being they have little choice but to resort to indirect ways to reassert their own control. Researchers tell us that young people have the highest rates of dropout from mental health services of any age group.[96] While this is sometimes presented as a sign of poor judgement or lack of commitment to their own well-being, it might be better understood as one of the few ways that young people have to express their resistance to decisions in which they have had no part — as the old saying goes, "they vote with their feet." Indeed, a number of the young people we spoke to about unhappy contacts with counsellors ended with the predictable refrain: "I didn't go back."

While some young people walk away from help, others are forced to exercise more subtle ways of resisting 'help' they have not chosen. It seemed in talking to young people, many had found ways of appearing to comply with the decisions of adults around them, while quietly upholding their own agency. One of the primary ways that young people are able to do this is through silent disengagement. As one young client of a school counselling service explained:

> I didn't really like it at first. I just sat there and refused to say anything. I was like I'm not doing this, I can't be bothered. So I just sat there and I was like "*No!*"[n]

Other young clients also told us how they appeared to go along with the session, while all the while carefully holding back on meaningful participation as one young client put it:

> I didn't say anything … I wouldn't say anything. I'd just sit there and listen to them and only give half of what needs to be said with one-word answers.[1]

As a psychologist, I have often been in a room with a young client who showed reluctance to engage in this way. In the past, I might have assumed that the young person was struggling to express themselves or was uncomfortable about talking to a stranger in this formal setting. I would have imagined that, as a 'good' psychologist, I should be able to draw them out and help them feel more comfortable to speak. However, after listening to the perspective of young clients I can more easily recognise this non-engagement as an attempt to claim back some kind of control from a situation in which a young person has been made to feel powerless; a legitimate assertion of their right to decide when they need help and what help they prefer.

The young people we spoke to also described how they continued to, quietly but determinedly, exercise their own power through the process of therapy. One young man who had been referred to a mental health service explained how he carefully monitored what he shared with the clinicians:

> Sometimes I'd control, well not control, but watch what I'd say … I guess it was a choice if I could say anything or not, but I just wasn't really in the mood to talk at all sort of thing, because being the fact that I didn't want to be there in the first place.[1]

This same young man went on to describe how he consciously refused to participate in the therapy as it continued:

> Yeah I was pretty quiet, didn't say anything. Every time they would say anything I was like "no that's wrong" sort of thing but I just kept it to myself.[1]

This kind of passive resistance extended not only to what young clients were willing to speak about in counselling but also to what they were prepared to listen to. As another of the young man who had attended therapy at a mental health service described:

> I would go in there, not really listen to what they have to say, because I had to be there. I had to be there, so I didn't really care about what they were trying to say.[l]

The word 'resistant' is often used in psychology and psychiatry to refer to those people who do not wish to follow the recommendations of professionals who are assumed to know what is best for them.[97] Framed in this way, there is little space for accepting the validity of a client's preference for a different approach to their mental health. This is perhaps true for all clients, but most especially for young clients, whose ideas about what they need or want are sometimes treated as irrational, irresponsible, and immature.[98]

While some young people described being robbed of their power in encounters with mental health professionals with little alternative but to submit or withdraw, we also heard many accounts of how young people had found more positive ways to exercise their agency in help-seeking and counselling.

Although the young people we spoke to had sometimes been frustrated by their inability to make decisions about what help they wanted, many still emphasised their own choice in selecting when they wanted to participate and which aspects, if any, of the counselling they were prepared to take on board. Many of the young clients we interviewed showed a high level of awareness and discernment about what approaches and ideas had worked well for them and those which they saw as less helpful. As one young woman who had used the counselling service at her school explained:

> I think it's important to know what works for you. I knew certain things that didn't really sit well with me and you just move on from that and maybe change or see someone else.[n]

The young people we spoke to also conveyed an astute understanding of their counsellors' strengths and weaknesses and how these fitted with their own needs and priorities. One young man explained how he had tried out several of the counsellors who worked at his school and how, knowing each of them, he would approach the one whose particular skills best suited his needs at any time:

> It depends on the situation you're in I guess. If it's girls … about girl issues a lot but I've gone to [Counselor 1] a lot because he knew more. I don't know, he's been through it all. He's older, he's wiser. But say if I was in trouble with guys giving me threats or something like that I know I'd go to [Counselor 2] because he knows the guys, … he can give me advice on how to get them to back off. If its family issues, which were happening a lot, I'd

> go to [Counselor 3] and would just be able to, she'd give me that retreat away from family.[n]

While most of the young people who discussed this seemed philosophical in the face of their counsellor's relative weaknesses, some offered the occasional rather unnerving assessment of their competence. One young client said, in a rather kindly tone, that she thought perhaps that counselling had been "the wrong job" for one of the less helpful counsellors she had seen. Another young person simply dismissed the, no doubt well-intentioned, suggestions of her counsellor and made it clear that she preferred to rely on her own sense of what worked for her:

> I don't really think that stuff works with me. I don't like being told to go for a walk or something. This is what I feel like when I'm angry or upset or something. I don't feel like drawing a picture or going for a walk. I just feel like sitting and having a cry … It's not what I want to do when I'm feeling like that.[n]

Of the young people we interviewed who had had positive experiences of counselling, many attributed this to their own abilities to take what they needed from counselling and to discard what was less helpful. Most of the young people we spoke to seemed to be actively evaluating what the counsellors could offer and weighing this against their own self-knowledge and preferences as one young woman explained:

> Well, I think it's really important that people don't rely on guidance because I found that I actually feel a lot better dealing with my life by myself sometimes. At the end of the day, I didn't take all their advice … I've been to counselling so many times. but at the end of the day I'm so straightforward and I'll just do what I feel at the time. It doesn't mean it's always a good thing, but I just do things without thinking, so sometimes I would structure a plan in counselling, but as soon as I leave the room it sort of, I'll go home and do what feels right I suppose.[n]

While this young person recognised that her decisions might not always be 'best' for her, she still felt strongly that in the end, she wanted to be the one to decide what she would do.

One of the most disconcerting insights I gained into young people's resistance to professional control during our interviews is that the professionals working with them were likely to have been largely unaware of how their efforts were missing the mark. One young woman told me a story about how her counsellor had advised her on how to manage a troubled relationship and sent her away from the session with a pamphlet containing information about healthy relationships which the young client did not think particularly relevant to her situation. She explained that as she left the session she threw the pamphlet in the nearest rubbish bin. When I asked what she had said to her counsellor, she replied that she had simply said "Thank you."[n]

There has been a growing awareness of the need for counsellors to listen to their clients' evaluation of sessions and outcomes. There are a range of measures and tools now specifically designed to tap into clients' ratings of their counselling.[99] But while these are well-intentioned it seems unlikely the power imbalances that impact on young clients would enable honest feedback in this form and a better strategy would be to create more space for young clients to be involved in determining the agenda and direction of their counselling experience.

Reclaiming agency: *You get to choose the direction in your life*

While many of the stories young people shared about their help-seeking reflected their disempowerment, we also heard very clearly about how young people felt far more willing to reach out for help when they were given the space to make their own choices. Being able to decide when they wanted to get help was very important. One insightful young client explained how being given a choice about whether or not to go to school counselling had been what finally helped her make this important decision for herself:

> I was at [the mental health service], and they recommended that I go to school counselling. At first I was like "Nah, no way!" Then my parents both said to me you can go on your own accord. You don't have to go just because *we* think it's a good idea. And everyone was recommending that I go there, but they were like it's up to you. So eventually I thought I'll just give it a go, and then I went there.[n]

We also heard a number of young people talking about counselling experiences where they felt respected and able to exercise their own agency. For the most part, it seemed that young people felt that they gained most from counselling when they were encouraged to explore their own experiences and to make decisions about their own lives, and we heard less mention of strategies they might have learnt to manage their mental health. One young woman explained how she valued the way she had been enabled to find her own answers through counselling:

> I sort of didn't want to go into counselling and hear something that I don't want to hear … It was helpful when they would sit down with me and say you get to choose the direction in your life … It's basically been good because I talked a lot, and even though I agreed with absolutely nothing my counsellor said, I came up with my own cool versions … Which was really good. You know, after talking about it, I kind of did make more sense of it out of my own mind. And just having, I mean she asked the right questions and she did. And I just didn't like the cool version she got. But in forcing me to think about those questions, I got a lot out of it.[n]

The idea that counselling, at its best, was not advice but rather operated as a sounding board for the clients' own self-discovery came up again and again in our conversations. One young woman contrasted her negative idea of counselling as being told what to do, with a good experience that she had had with another counsellor who created a space for her to find her own answers:

> … I scheduled another appointment. But not with the same counsellor. And that was less like "counselling." She wasn't really like telling me what I should do and stuff like that. It was more me talking about it and her helping me to expand on what I was thinking. And that was really helpful.[n]

When counselling accommodates young people's need for agency, they are more able to use it as a refuge from other relationships in which they feel judged and pressured to respond in certain ways. One young person gave this account of a counsellor who had given her a unique space in which she had the freedom to think about her own choices:

> A lot of the times when I would try to tell my parents or tell my friends what was happening, they are very quick to say, "This is what you should do." I didn't have anyone that would just step back and just actually listen.[n]

It is clear that young people want to be respected and to have collaborative relationships with their counsellors in which they can be active in deciding what matters to them. All of this points to the importance of allowing young people to exercise their agency and for professionals to show respect for their ideas and opinions during the process of supporting them. While most models of therapy would have little difficulty in allowing that a mutually respectful relationship between client and counsellor is more likely to be productive than a hierarchical one, this requires a little more thought and attention to actualise within a therapeutic relationship with a young client.[100] Cognitive Behaviour Therapy, for example, strongly advocates a collaborative partnership between the counsellor and client when working on the client's difficulties. Nonetheless, common strategies such a 'homework' can evoke unpleasant associations with school and position the young client back in the role of a student with its resonances of the classroom situation.[101] Similarly, the 'Socratic questioning' style that is intended to help the client challenge their own thinking may be experienced in much the same way as the questioning teachers use when they know the answer but want to check that their student does. It may be useful to think of working with a young client as being like working with those clients who have experienced ongoing forms of disempowerment, such as abuse, throughout their lives.[102] In these cases, professionals have to remain highly attuned to power dynamics and ensure that their clients retain a sense of control over the therapy.

The need for young people to have their right to agency recognised extends beyond the counselling room, and many told us how they saw recovery from mental health problems as part of a self-development process which ultimately they directed themselves. When we spoke to a group of young people who had come through a period of dealing with quite significant mental health problems, they emphasised the importance of not relying on others. As one explained:

> I think that a lot of people in mental health system rely too much on other people for things and they really need to stop that attitude … People can't do the work for you.[k]

Becoming well, in fact, was seen by some young people as being synonymous with being able to reclaim their own agency and overcome feelings of disempowerment that they associated with being unwell:

> I feel a lot more in control of my life and what I can do. I never had any of that growing up. I didn't have any autonomy so for my personality in particular, I really need that … I'm very much my own person.[k]

Respect for the agency of young people is not only important for their willingness to engage with therapy but the experience of agency is also seen by them as an important marker of their recovery from mental health problems.

One of the attractions of digital spaces for young people is because it is an arena in which they can exercise their own agency without the scrutiny of the adults around them. In talking with young people, we were told about how many of their online practices were specifically designed to allow them privacy from the adults in their lives. Ito and her colleagues, who completed a large research study on young people's use of digital technology in the United States, described how these online spaces allow young people to evade the adult oversight that is so much a part of young people's lives today.[103] While engagement with digital technology allows young people greater opportunity to exercise their own agency outside the physical restraints of family or school, ironically, these same freedoms highlight the contradictions between this cyber-freedom and the constraints that continue to govern the everyday lives of young people.

Given the challenges that young people face in seeking help in the offline world, it is no wonder that they often prefer to seek help in online spaces. For them, the internet represents a space where they can choose the help they prefer and where whatever decisions they make are unlikely to result in an adult taking control of their lives.

When we interviewed young people about their preferences for online and offline support, we heard a great deal about the barriers that prevented them from looking for face-to-face support and many of these related to potential threats to their agency. In contrast, one of the aspects that drew them to digital support was the greater freedom it allowed. When we spoke to young people about the use of a text-based counselling service, their ability to retain control of the experience and avoid unnecessary intrusion by adults was a highly valued aspect of this mode of support. One young person who had used this service, for example, explained how, in contrast to face-to-face counselling, they appreciated the option to close down the encounter when they chose:

> So I just like texting and like, I can just open up when I am texting and I will be like okay: "I need to close the door now."[j]

If text counselling allows young clients to experience some degree of freedom, engaging with peers or online resources allows even more agency. In interviews focused on their online help-seeking, it was clear that for many this was a preference over face-to-face engagement precisely because it allowed them greater agency to choose when they wanted to reach out, who they wanted to confide in and how much or how little they wanted to say. One participant spoke about valuing how her online support seeking practices allowed her to move at her own pace:

> I think a lot of young people would be quite hesitant to speak to someone in person - the way I see it is it's a bigger step to initiate going to a counselling service than it is to look up resources in your own time and pace.[d]

The anonymity enabled by some online support seeking helped to provide a sense of protection from unwelcome intrusion and even when it was not anonymous, the feeling of distance created by being behind a screen also helped young people to retain a sense that they could make their own decisions.

Attempts to engage young people with support need to take account of their relative powerlessness and the importance they assign to their agency. In order to reach young people, it is important to provide them with choices and facilitate, rather than direct, their recovery.

What do young people want?

Young people want their agency to be respected when they engage with support. They want to be able to make choices about when and from whom they seek help. When they engage with counsellors they want to have the space to express and explore their own priorities and to work with someone who will support them on the journey they wish to take.

Those working with young people can help them by

- Respecting their choices about when and whether to ask for help.
- Treating them as equals in the process of providing mental health support.
- Providing facilitative spaces, including online spaces, in which they can make their own decisions.
- Supporting them on their chosen journey towards adulthood.

6 Relationships and mental health: *You only share things with those you trust*

There is a particularly compelling cartoon that has young people walking down the street staring at their phones. The tag reads: 'The zombie apocalypse is here.' This representation of young people is obviously meant to be amusing but also highlights one of the consistent worries that adults raise about young people today: their apparent disconnection from 'real' social interaction. With young people immersing themselves in the digital world, parents and other adults are understandably concerned that they might be missing out on the advantages of social connection in their lives and that this will have a negative effect on their mental health.

Almost every book about how to ensure good mental health will contain a reference to the value of social support and the negative impacts of isolation. Social connection has long been recognised as powerful protection against depression and suicidality and as an antidote to stress and other kinds of adversity.[104] A trusting relationship with a counsellor is also widely viewed as a key ingredient in the effectiveness of psychological therapies, with some researchers arguing it is more important than any particular technical strategy.[105] If it is true that young people are no longer forming good social relationships, from a psychological perspective this would indeed be a concern, with potential to affect their well-being as well as their capacity to benefit from professional support.

But in our conversations with young people, we heard consistently about how important good relationships were in their lives. Confronted by the alienating and individualising impacts of neoliberalism, young people appeared to be actively seeking out belonging and connection but perhaps finding it in places and ways that are less familiar to the adults around them.

To understand this generation, we need to know what it is that they want from their relationships and where, and how they find this. Furthermore, if we want to be able to support young people in distress, we will need to find out what kinds of relationships they want with mental health services and the professionals who work there.

Trusting in friendship: *Like when you are deep friends*

When young people talk about relationships, it is most often their peer friendships that take priority. One of the stereotypes about young people is social

DOI: 10.4324/9780429322457-6

media, where friends can be made by tapping on a screen and friend groups often number in the hundreds, has diluted the meaning of friendship. But, interestingly, the young people we spoke to were very clear that they were not just looking for these kinds of 'friends' but rather for more meaningful connections. One young man articulated his understanding of the difference between social media 'friends' and real friends:

> Like you would probably see that, particularly on say a site like Tumblr in which a lot of the people following a certain blog or something is not the same. You don't know them. They don't know you. They are not friends. They are not close friends as you would have 400 people on Facebook. They could be anybody.[b]

In contrast with these apparently indiscriminate networks, he and other young people seemed to be searching for a sense of intimacy and real connection that could only be developed over time. One young woman gave an account of how 'real' friendships were developed, recognising a gradual process of getting to know someone and developing a sense of connection to them:

> The more intimate you are with someone relationship wise, like the more you trust someone and the more like when you are deep friends with someone then in a sense you become attached to them. I feel like once you become attached to someone then you care about them more and when they say something like that it matters to you more. Whereas if it's like some acquaintance like you just added on Facebook it will be like "Oh okay."[a]

The young people we spoke to were very discerning in their understanding of different kinds of friendship. For example, they explained the importance of being able to distinguish between different 'levels' of friends, from those who might be better described as acquaintances to those who they might hang out with at school or on the weekend, right down to the, usually small group of friends in whom they confided.

The development of trust emerged as a key ingredient in young people's friendships — in both their online and offline worlds. While trust might always have been regarded as a valuable part of friendship, it seems that the current generation, with fewer rules and institutional norms to guide them, takes increasing responsibility to make sure their worlds are safe. They may be more conscious than other generations of the potential for breaches of trust of privacy and loyalty. Trust emerged again and again as a theme through our interviews with youth. For young people, trust needed to be developed slowly and cautiously as this high school student told us:

> Yeah, with like trust, you like do something, you tell them something and then if they kind of follow through with that and they don't tell anyone then you trust them a bit more and then it slowly builds up and up and up.[a]

Young people seem to be very aware of the importance of having clear rules about trust in relationships. For example, one young woman who was a member of a tight-knit friend group explained how they felt comfortable sharing secrets within this group, safe in the knowledge that it would go no further:

> We know that if we tell one person something the whole group of seven of us is gonna find out but also know that no one else will find out. We trust our group and it will stick to our group. But no one else.[a]

Unsurprisingly, given these requirements, we heard stories about the harsh retribution, even ostracism, meted out to young people who broke the sacred rules of trust.

In contrast to concerns that many adults have about lack of privacy and safety on the internet, trust featured as significantly, if not more so, in online interactions than in face-to-face friend groups. When I spoke to young people about their social media use I was surprised by the priority that young people gave this. In one study where I interviewed young people via WhatsApp instant messaging to find out how they gave and received support on social media, they emphasised how important it was for them to feel 'safe' before they were willing to talk openly about themselves or their lives. One young woman, for example, explained how she would only use a Facebook group with a small group of friends to talk about very personal issues:

> It's like a safe space for young people to be open about their life but in a restrictive manner where only the friends they trust can see this.[i]

The message was clear for both online and offline friendships, as one young person succinctly put it:

> You only share things with those you trust.[i]

During our discussions with young people about their social media use, we heard a great deal not only about the value of their connections to friend groups but also, interestingly, about the way that people experienced a sense of connection with others in anonymous online groups. We heard, from both young men and women, for example, about the way they saw these groups as an opportunity to make friends online, even where these friends remained nameless and faceless. Some described a growing sense of connection to others in these anonymous online spaces with trust developing slowly over time.

Rather than basing friendship on shared activities, the young people we spoke to saw friendship as fundamentally about caring. One young person explained that this was the most important thing in her life:

> I mean I've got people that care for me, that love me for who I am. Regardless of whichever situation I am going through they are always going to be there for me.[b]

The idea that people should care for one another was not always as clearly articulated but seemed to be a common thread that ran through many of our conversations with young people. While this circle of care could include family or other adults, most often young people thought of their similar-aged friends as being the ones who mattered. Young people today are clear that friends are not simply the people they 'hang out' with, go to parties with, or play rugby with. Friends, for young people, were those people who they could count on to be there for them.

In addition to having trust and care as a basis for friendship, young people also prioritised understanding and acceptance from their friends. In opposition to pressures to match up to social expectations of themselves, they were looking for spaces in which they did not have to protect their image or pretend to be someone that they were not. I first heard the word 'relatable' in my conversations with young people, although I have heard about it in many places since. This word, which has gained increasing currency among young people, is used to describe the way that young people can see themselves in characters or situations. Relatability is also used sometimes to describe the kind of camaraderie that can develop between young people to share intimate and sometimes embarrassing experiences with one another.[106] The young people we spoke to seem to have adapted the concept to mean some mixture of these: a sense of shared experience that allowed them to drop their façade, enabled them to step away from the pressures that they experienced in their lives, and find a space where they would not be judged. This was particularly important for young people when they were feeling vulnerable or distressed. Those we spoke to provided many examples of this and how they had been comforted by sharing with peers who could connect to their experiences. As one of the high school students we interviewed put it:

> 'Cause I think it's like the fear of being judged is why like guys don't really talk to each other about stuff. Once you realise that they're all going through the same stuff that you are, then you feel you can like open up to them more, so yeah.[a]

This highly prized relatability that young people experienced with intimate friends occurred less often with the adults around them. Many young people spoke about how they felt adults did not understand their world. One young person, for example, explained why young people were reluctant to talk to adults about sensitive issues like distress:

> I think there is a certain perception that adults don't understand, that they are out of touch, that they are not relatable, that they don't understand.[b]

Interestingly, the notion of relatability seemed to apply as much to institutions and organisations as it did to people. Ubiquitous advertising on social media means that young people are exposed to a continuous stream of what we know as 'spam.' As with friendships, they have developed a sophisticated ability to distinguish between genuine and honest, or false and manipulative, messages. As one young person explained, it was important for professional mental health messages to come from a trustworthy or relatable institution if young people were going to engage with them:

> ... these things are kind of seen as a big outside quite corporate thing, quite foreign coming in and it's just, it seems quite intimidating, it's not relatable and so for a lot of people in kind of small communities, it's just alienating.[d]

While trust, care, and relatability seemed to be common concerns among the young people we spoke to, there was also an acknowledgement that some young people might do friendship differently. There was, for example, an awareness that boys and girls wanted different things from their friends as one young man said about his group of male friends:

> they're there for their mates and stuff but it just feels different.[a]

While boys and young men tended to rather just 'hang out,' girls and young women shared more personal and emotionally laden issues with one another. There were some exceptions, however, and it was encouraging to hear from one male high school student about how he and his friends regularly went camping together and sitting around the fire at night had made it a habit to speak openly with one another about how they were feeling.

Despite many differences between young people, it was clear that friendships mattered enormously to this digital generation. While it may be that friendships do not matter *more* to young people than to their parents and grandparents, there may be added pressures in their hyperawareness of the potential for breaches of trust and the importance of establishing safety in these relationships. The priority that young people assign to relationships offers both opportunities and challenges for professionals and services to connect with them.

Needing connection: *No one feels comfortable talking to a stranger*

For young people, the development of intimacy and trust in a relationship with someone who they feel can understand them is central to their being able to talk about personal issues.[107] It is hardly surprising then, that from the perspective of a young person, talking to someone about distress or a mental health problem could only happen in the context of a safe relationship, a requirement other researchers have also emphasised.[108]

The relationship between a client and counsellor, sometimes called a 'working alliance,' is recognised in the professional literature as vital to being able to work successfully with a client in therapy.[109] But while mental health professionals are aware of the importance of this relationship, it is probably fair to say that there is rather more focus on professional training on skills and strategies for bringing about change. Counsellors and other mental health professionals do recognise the importance of safety in the counselling relationship but generally see this as being provided by professionalism, confidentiality, and neutrality. For young people, however, it seems that their expectations of a counsellor were closer to what they expected in their friendships more generally; a relationship in which intimacy was able to be developed in the context of trust, genuine care, and relatability.

When we spoke to young people about their ideas about counselling, it was abundantly clear there needed to be a strong sense of connection before a young client would discuss their problems with a counsellor. As one young person put it:

> Cause no one feels comfortable talking to a stranger about your problems...' Cause when you actually know the person you know that they genuinely care. 'Cause otherwise they'll be like I don't personally know you...[n]

When young people told stories about their experiences with a school counsellor, they spoke about a careful process of getting to know their counsellor before they would be willing to share important information. Many young clients told us about 'holding back' until they felt sure that the person they were talking to was someone they could trust. While this seems to be an entirely appropriate way of approaching a new relationship, it is often at odds with the way that mental health professionals are trained to conduct their first sessions with a client. The emphasis for mental health clinicians is often on getting enough information about the client's problems through these first sessions. They are under pressure to be able to determine any immediate risks, to understand their client's problem, and to plan the best course of treatment within the first few meetings. But some of the young people we spoke to had been surprised and alarmed at being asked intensely personal questions in their first counselling session. Others spoke about how they had appreciated those counsellors who had given them some time to feel safe and comfortable before expecting them to speak about the things that were worrying them, as one young client described:

> [My counsellor] didn't make me feel uncomfortable, didn't make me go straight into everything I was feeling and stuff, she kind of just talked about me and what I liked to do and just my hobbies and everything and then would just make little jokes with me so I'd like loosen up and laugh with her.[n]

Given that some of the young people who experience mental health problems are likely to have a history of relationship problems — experiences of being let down, abused, or abandoned — the expectation that they should immediately feel comfortable to make themselves vulnerable to a stranger seems especially inappropriate.[110] One young person who had been referred to a mental health service told us how her past experiences had made it especially difficult for her to trust her counsellor:

> Before I went to [the mental health service] I wasn't good at opening up to people that I didn't know at all and so I thought I don't want to sit there and talk about my life problems when I don't know someone.[l]

Young people have a clear expectation that the opportunity to develop a sense of connection with a counsellor must come first before they would be willing to talk to them about things that mattered. They also recognised that it took time to develop a more trusting relationship with someone with whom they felt comfortable to share their vulnerability. There were many touching accounts from young people about how they had gradually, over time, come to know their counsellor and started to feel safe. One young person captured the way she and her counsellor had formed a connection:

> I feel like I got to know her sort of or she got to know me, and I think that was quite important.[l]

But while some young people had experienced the comfort of developing a relationship with a counsellor, slowly and in their own time, the mental health services are not always well-set-up to accommodate this. There is increased pressure on services to offer short-term interventions — the justification being that usually they are efficient and have a strong evidence base. But in addition to this, there are strong economic and institutional pressures also driving the increased reliance on short-term models of treatment.[111] While these interventions can be helpful for some people, for others struggling with long-term and serious problems they can be grossly inadequate.[112] It is also clear that this model of short-term intervention may not be a particularly good fit for the relational needs of young people who respond better when they can connect to a person slowly over a period of time. One young person who had struggled with ongoing mental health problems articulated her frustration in being unable to connect to her counsellor in the brief time available:

> Who is to say that in six sessions I am going to even be able to build enough of a relationship with a person to even begin to talk about this kind of shit? That always really fucked me off.[k]

There are also other ways in which mental health services do not meet the relational needs of young people. In many child and adolescent services, professionals work in teams where they may share a load of a single client across a number of different clinicians. In some cases, there might be two mental health professionals who conduct the initial assessment and another who is assigned the therapy. If the client is especially lucky they may see the assigned therapist for 12 weeks of therapy. If the young person needs to return for any reason, however, they might go through the same process with different people and different faces, often asking the same questions and making the same recommendations. Young people's frustration with this aspect of the mental health services was a continuous refrain in our interviews. One young person captured the futility she felt at having this experience again and again:

> it was again kind of the same story around... I think within the first three appointments I saw six different people ... every time I see someone, it is always a different person.[k]

The services in New Zealand and many other countries also make a clear differentiation between adult and child services, with an age cut off that means a young person may need to move abruptly from one service to another.[18] This can be very disruptive and frightening for a young person. One young client spoke about how the support she had been receiving through a social service agency stopped suddenly at the age of 17:

> Coming out of [an organisation's] care was pretty intense. Like, they kind of just, like kick you out–see you later, good luck sort of thing and I needed a little more support than that. Normal 17 year-olds don't move out at 17–it is not a normal way to move out.[k]

For those young people who are lucky enough to be able to find and establish a good ongoing relationship with a counsellor, the relationship inevitably ended as they reached the cut-off age. Some young people approached their therapy with understandable caution as a result of this:

> It's not good to become too attached though, because um, when I end up finishing at [the mental health service], which they reckon won't be for another year, I don't want to be like too attached to [counsellor] and rely on her a lot.[l]

While a relationship with a GP or dentist may last for decades, there is an irony in the fact that mental health services, which require a real emotional connection between practitioners and clients, tend to work with discrete episodes of care and disconnections between services.

For young people to feel comfortable in counselling, it was also very important for them to find the 'right' person to talk to. In contrast to adults who might prioritise the qualifications, reputation, and success rate of a counsellor in their choice, the young people we spoke to seemed largely oblivious to these external trappings of professionalism and authority. Instead, they seemed more concerned with whether the person they spoke to was friendly, relatable, and kind. Those we spoke to who had had a positive experience with a counsellor described an intuitive process of feeling that someone was 'right' for them. One young person was clear that without this the therapy process could not be expected to work:

> You just need to be able to click with them as a person and if you can't click with them then it's not gonna help you.[b]

While not all young people were looking for the same qualities in a counsellor, there did seem to be some characteristics that appeared commonly in their accounts of more helpful encounters with mental health professionals. Overall, the young people we spoke to seemed to prefer counsellors who were informal in their style and more 'relatable' to youth. One of the younger people who took part in our study of school counselling, for example, described a counsellor she had connected well to, like this:

> He was quite laid back. He kind of acted like a teenager at some points. He wouldn't mind swearing or anything. It made me think okay this guy, he knows how to relate sort of thing. I didn't want to feel like I was talking to some snobby professor or something like that. Just someone who I could actually chat with.[n]

Rather than seeing 'professionalism' as an asset, some young people found mental health professionals who presented themselves in this way as cold and difficult to connect to. In fact, a number of those we spoke to used the word 'professional' exclusively as a criticism of some counsellors they had seen in the past. One young person provided an example of the difficulty she had in talking to a clinician who was very business-like in her approach:

> With the first psychiatrist, she was quite a bit older, so I found it quite hard to talk to her, and she was very formal, and she would sit down and be like "now when was the last time that you self-harmed" and it was just really straight to the point questions, and it was sort of, I didn't feel like I got to know her or she got to know me.[l]

Young people were looking for something beyond title or competence, for something that simply felt "nice" and "comfortable." For some young people, there was an automatic sense of connection to younger clinicians who they felt shared their worldview, but even when the counsellor was older, they seemed to find a connection in an attitude of warmth and relatability. One young person described his slightly older counsellor like this:

> She was just really bubbly, cute as well in a way for an old person. She just spoke nicely like she was funny and stuff and she just, I think she was overall like a really caring, nice person.[n]

In addition, part of what seems to help young people connect with a counsellor was a sense that the relationship with the counsellor was reciprocal. Typically, the relationship between a counsellor and their client is one-sided, where the client reveals themselves and the counsellor responds neutrally and with minimal self-disclosure.[113] But in our interviews, young people made it clear that they wanted to know the counsellor was a person who actually cared and that they too were gaining something from the time they spent with their client. Young people described how they wanted to know who the counsellor was as a person and appreciated it when some counsellors had revealed aspects of themselves. This kind of disclosure from the counsellor — either through telling things about themselves or showing aspects of themselves in the counselling room — seemed to make it easier for young people to find the 'relatability' they were looking for, as the following account of counselling given by a young client suggests:

> He's actually told me things like who he is and his personality and he brings the conversation to relate to it and that so it just helps ... he knows what I'm going through. He has a similarity so it's good. It's not someone who has no clue.[n]

Many of the accounts the young people gave us of counselling experiences that had not gone well highlighted their fears that a counsellor might not be trying to establish an authentic relationship. One young woman, for example, gave this critical account of previous mental health professionals she had seen:

> The others were just I think very much into their job so they were more focused on I guess what they have to do and get it done.[n]

In contrast to this, young people seemed to value counsellors who made it clear that they themselves were taking something from their encounter with the client and those who appeared genuinely interested in their clients:

> She'll say, 'I really enjoy our talks and I really want to catch up with you in the future,' you know, because she asks about my life and how I'm doing, not just about my problems. When she asks me about my life I know she's genuinely asking me because she's interested.[n]

This idea that the counsellor was really trying to understand them and wanted to know what mattered to them was also really important as one young woman who had had a good experience of mental health services explained:

> It kind of felt as if they were listening to you with the intent to understand, not just the intent to reply. You know like they were really understanding. Yeah they really wanted to try and just get to know you as a person.[l]

In addition to genuinely wanting to know about them, young people expressed the hope that their counsellors might genuinely care for them. One young woman explained how, in spite of being aware that her psychologist saw other clients, she wanted to believe that she had a special relationship with her:

> It feels good that, it feels like, I mean I know that there's lot of other people that care about me, but at least one person that cares about me. And I don't know if she does it with, I don't know how many clients or people she has, I mean it's … quite heartfelt, it's quite good and it's nice to know that, out of all the people that she does, she also remembers you. I mean it's as if you are the only client, if you know what I mean. She makes everyone like that.[1]

The thought that a counsellor simply saw one client and moved on to the next seemed unacceptable to the young people we spoke to, who were looking for that a sense that they mattered, uniquely, to their counsellor:

> It just kind of felt like your problems weren't really, you were just another client they were seeing you know, that would come in and you would spill your guts out to them about everything that was happening and then they would move on to the next person. There was something really impersonal and it didn't feel right.[1]

When young people spoke about good counselling relationships, these were often described as being very much like the sort of friendship they might enjoy with their peers. One young woman who had seen two different clinicians at a mental health service articulated explicitly how she had felt more able to connect with a counsellor who spoke to her as a 'friend' rather than as a professional:

> With one counsellor I just connected with her instantly and with the other not so much. The one talks to me like I'm her friend or something, and the other talks to me as if he's my counsellor kind of thing.[1]

Many professionals have been doubtful about the ability of text and other online forms of counselling to provide young people with a relational connection. But, as with young people's engagement with one another on social media, it was clear that the relationship also mattered a great deal in online counselling.

When we interviewed young people about their experience of using the online text counselling service offer by Youthline in New Zealand, we were surprised to hear that many of the clients had felt that they had been able to build a relationship with a counsellor in spite of the anonymity of the interaction and the absence of visual or auditory cues. We heard for example about how young people felt they came to 'know' the person they communicated with via text. One young person described how, in spite of the limits of text communication, she experienced the anonymous counsellor as a 'person':

> It's not like a text, but she's like a person... It's a person like she's kind of like um my, like my sibling or someone from my family the way she talked.[j]

Young people's ability to find a relational connection via text with someone they did not know and could not see might reflect their familiarity and comfort with digital communication. However, it also seemed that some young people's need to find a relationship was so strong that they were able to find this even in anonymous interactions. One young woman gave us a very interesting account of how she had texted the counselling service because she was distressed by a tussle between her boyfriend and her mother in which she felt caught in the middle. It was exam time and her mother wanted her to stay at home and study, but her boyfriend wanted her to see him and felt she should take a stand against her mother. Her text conversation took place over two days with two different, anonymous counsellors. When asked who she felt she had been speaking to in the first text counselling interaction, she gave this description:

> Yeah, just something made it feel like it was a guy. Yeah, he actually seemed like he cared. Yeah, so it was sort of, I think that's why it felt like it was my boyfriend, because even though my boyfriend didn't want to talk to me, this person seemed like what I wanted my boyfriend to be doing.[j]

When we asked her later about the second counsellor, she explained that she thought this was a woman, someone perhaps closer to her mother's age. While we do not know the precise cues that informed the image of her counsellors, it seemed likely that these were in some way influenced by her own needs in this situation. A young man who would be like her boyfriend, only more understanding, and an older woman who perhaps could give her mother's perspective. This example suggests that young people may be able to conjure the kind of relationship they need, using only minimal cues in digital encounters.

The relatability that we had heard so much about during interviews about friendship and face-to-face encounters with counsellors was also described as important in text counselling by the young people we spoke to. One young client who had used the text counselling service, for example, explained how she had reached the conclusion that the counsellor she was talking to was young like herself and how important this was for her:

> Cause what they told us is that some people at Youthline, most of them are our age. And I mention what is happening and they have an idea, they get what's wrong. That's the good thing. That's why I kind of trusted them because I knew that they would be in our generation and stuff.[j]

This story also highlights one of the other significant challenges to the client's ability to establish a relationship with a counsellor; while a client may continue a text counselling conversation for hours or days, they are likely to have to engage with several different counsellors who are working in shifts. Strangely, however, this seemed to pose less of a problem to the young clients we spoke to than might have been expected. One young client explained, for example, how she was aware that her text counsellors had swapped shifts over the period that she was talking to them but her experience was that the connection she felt with the first counsellor flowed over into the next interaction:

> Yeah, I kind of had a thought that this probably isn't the same person. But they sort of understood like the other person did. And so there was still that feeling of comfort and trust that I had with the other person. Yeah so it was quite good.[j]

It was also noticeable how the clients of the text counselling services sometimes talked about their counsellor as 'they.' While sometimes this phrase is used for people of non-binary gender identity, in this context it seemed to be a way of talking about more than one counsellor as though somehow they were part of a composite entity:

> I thought at the time it was the same person. And they really thought, they know how I was feeling. They were like my friends, like how they get worried with you, so they text you back right away. It made me feel that way.[j]

In some cases, we heard how this sense of connection seemed to extend to the organisation as a whole. One young person spoke, for example, about how he saw Youthline as being like a "guardian angel" who watched over him.

Even with the anonymity of text counselling where interactions were reliant on short text messages without any sense of who the counsellor was and no verbal communication to convey their understanding and acceptance, young people seemed to be able to find a strong sense of connection.

Relying on professionalism: *I put my trust in them*

While the relationship that young people were looking for with a counsellor seemed in many ways to be similar to a friendship, there were ways in which young people recognised some important areas of difference. While trust in friendships was seen as very important it was not always guaranteed. The obligation to maintain trust in the form of confidentiality is a particular priority for young people.[114] While the word 'professional' was usually used in a derogatory way, young people did appear to still value and expect some aspects of professional behaviour in their counsellors.

Confidentiality emerged as a priority in all of our interviews with young people who had made use of some sort of mental health support. Many of the young people we spoke to explained that this guarantee of privacy was a major part of the appeal of taking a problem to a counsellor rather than simply talking to a friend. As one young person put it:

> The counsellor was like out of the situation - didn't know my mum, and I knew it would be confidential I felt and everything which was good.[n]

Although counsellors and other professionals usually work within a clear ethical obligation to hold confidentiality, young people often raised concerns about whether they would adhere to this. We heard some stories that suggested that young people's concerns about potential breaches of confidentiality might have had a foundation in reality with examples of situations in which a counsellor had apparently revealed information about a young client to their parents or other teachers in a school setting. While there were, no doubt, cases in which this was done in the young person's best interests, for the young people we spoke to this was seen as an unacceptable threat to sense of safety as one young woman recounted:

> I think I had an issue where she might have called my mum at one point which it's meant to be confidential. I'm not sure if she called my mum but I remember finding her business card in my mum's drawer and I remember saying to my mum what is going on ... so I assumed she'd rung and told my mum so I didn't have much trust in her.[n]

When confidentiality was established this became part of a developing sense of safety in the relationship with the counsellor. One young woman described how she had started off feeling anxious about whether she could trust her counsellor, but slowly began to feel that this was a safe relationship, and an important part of that safety was the promise of confidentiality. Although initially, she found it difficult to open up in therapy, she gradually felt more able to talk about her problems:

> I just ended up trusting [the clinician] 'cause I thought she's not going to be mean, and she's not going to go tell anyone cause it's all confidential. Yeah, I just put all my trust in them.[l]

In addition to confidentiality, young people spoke about how a counsellor offered them a relationship outside of their normal life where they would not be judged. Some of the young people we spoke to recognised how these qualities could not always be guaranteed in friendship and found some reassurance that counsellors were expected to be neutral and accepting:

> It was just like my own time where I could talk about anything that I wanted and they wouldn't go off and tell the girl that they saw walking around in school, sort of like what friends do sometimes. It was really nice to know that I have that comfort with them, but also that they were there to help me and they won't just stare at me and be like: "You're weird."[l]

We also heard about how young people found a sense of relief in being able to talk to someone where they did not have to worry about the listener's feelings and whether what they said would be a burden on them. This quality of counselling seemed to provide a kind of refuge for young people, outside of the social pressures of their normal life. As one young person put it:

> Because like they won't get hurt with what you're saying or like get offended by it. If I talked to my mum then like she might be upset to see that I'm upset because you know I didn't want to upset her anymore. Yeah it's just easier to talk to a stranger, well not a stranger but just someone else.[n]

One of the other aspects of the counselling relationship which young people recognised as different to other relationships in their lives was the power that counsellors were able to exercise on their behalf. Unlike friends, mental health professionals were able to stand up for the young person, sometimes against the power of other adults in their lives. School counsellors, for example, were seen as important potential allies to young people in the context of an institution in which they have very little power to determine their choices. One young person explained how her school counsellor had helped to negotiate with teachers on her behalf and help them to be more sympathetic to her difficulties:

> I guess sometimes the teachers didn't really understand my stuff and I had someone to back me up … [My counsellor] would either go talk to them or email them and it helped me get to my classes because my teachers, the more they started understanding it and kind of treating me a bit differently than they did, the more I was happier to go to class because I knew that they were understanding and on board.[n]

Another young person explained how her counsellor had intervened to stop a situation in which she was being bullied:

> If I said someone in my class is saying horrible things to me she would say, 'do you want me to email the teacher and ask if you can move?' … like I prefer to sit up the back in the class because I don't like people looking. So, she'll email the teacher and ask to have me moved and sitting with a friend in the class.[n]

While young people might find it easier to disclose difficulties to a friend, they are aware that adults would have power to intervene more effectively, to advise them or protect them against issues like abuse. One young woman described her relief when she was finally able to disclose to her counsellor about the abuse she had been struggling with for a long time:

> I never told an adult about it, so finally an adult actually knew what has happened and stuff. It was kind of a weight off my shoulder because adults can obviously do more than teenagers can, so it was kind of like finding someone who can help to actually make a difference.[n]

Although the young people we spoke to seemed to be looking for a counselling relationship that more closely resembled a friendship than a professional service, they valued some of the assurances and protections that a professional relationship might offer, including confidentiality and the access to an adult who could advocate on their behalf.

In a world where young people can feel disconnected, relationships hold great importance. Relationships with peers remain central to young people's lives and are held to the highest standards of trust and authenticity. Similarly, young people cannot easily think of mental health support as occurring outside of these requirements for a good relationship. For young people today, it matters that they have a real relationship with a counsellor, one who is 'relatable,' genuinely cares about them and is trustworthy. These criteria appear to hold for both offline and online engagement with support.

What do young people want?

Young people want to have a relationship with a counsellor who is relatable, genuine, caring as well as professional. They want to have the opportunity to develop trust and safety in this relationship before they talk about the things that worry them.

Those working with young people can help by

- Recognising the importance that relationships have in their lives.
- Giving them time to get to know you.
- Providing them with trustworthy and safe relationships.
- Being genuine and 'real' in their relationships with young clients.
- Offering the assurance of confidentiality and professionalism.

7 Access and mental health: *It's there when you need it*

Difficulties with access to mental health care is often noted as one of the primary barriers to young people's using professional help. When this is discussed, researchers and service providers often refer to physical access and the constraints that young people might have in being able to travel to, or afford to see, a counsellor in their local area.[115] However, access is a broader issue; it not only does involve these practical considerations but also concerns more subtle elements that influence whether young people feel that professional help is easily available to them and whether they feel comfortable using it. Issues of access include the location of the services, the ease with which young people can make contact and arrange appointments, the degree to which they feel welcomed into these services, and whether they feel at ease in the space.

Existing mental health services for young people are often designed using models that were originally intended for adults. Many of these services are attached to hospitals or clinics and often require a formal referral from a doctor or teacher. Sessions usually happen at set times, booked in advance on a weekly basis, and last for a set amount of time.

Counselling services are based on models that have largely been unchanged for decades, but the world in which young people live today is very different. In spite of the constraints that continue to operate on their agency, young people have been led to expect greater freedom to choose and, being exposed to a wide array of ideas through the internet, they have a clearer sense of their preferences and the limits on the choices offered to them. In addition, having 24-hour access to communication on digital media from the comfort of their own bedrooms changes the way that young people think about space and time and their expectations of being able to reach someone when they are distressed. It is important to understand what gets in the way of young people being able to access support at the time they need it and what needs to change to ensure that young people can get this.

Finding a safe place: *An environment where I felt comfortable*

There is a long history of research showing that the way physical spaces are organised in mental health services and institutions will have a considerable impact

DOI: 10.4324/9780429322457-7

on people's experiences of themselves and others.[116] Buildings can be designed to produce different sorts of feelings. Large monument-type buildings induce feelings of awe for authority and increase a sense of our own insignificance; high-tech hospital buildings help to increase our faith in science and medicine, and small cottage-like spaces conjure up a sense of home. But we need to understand how buildings and spaces can be made more comfortable and friendly for young people when they are feeling distressed and vulnerable. To be able to engage young people with support, it is important to understand how different sorts of spaces might make it easier or more difficult for young clients to seek help and feel they can talk openly about personal issues.

In one of our studies, which looked at young people's first experience of a mental health assessment, participants told us that some of their initial fears had centred on how they imagined the physical characteristics of the mental health service. For young people, one of their few models for talking to adults about their difficulties is doctors' consulting rooms, which can feel cold and clinical and may be filled with intimidating medical equipment. This latter association is particularly likely to be at the forefront of young people's imaginations as, very often, these mental health services are actually located in hospital or health clinic settings. One young man described how when he had been told he was due to attend a mental health assessment at a hospital he had imagined something like his previous doctor's visits:

> And they just took me. I didn't know what it was. And I thought it was some medical thing 'cause we went to the hospital… I thought I was getting a check-up or something, but yeah it was that. I thought it was a check-up like a medical check-up thing.[m]

In this same study, several of the young people had been referred for a mental health assessment after some problem behaviour had resulted in an encounter with the youth justice service. For this group of young people, their expectation of the mental health service was understandably shaped by their previous experiences of police stations and other legal encounters. One young person imagined that the mental health service would look a lot like the setting of a television police show:

> I thought it was like, you know how you have police interviews, I thought it was going to be like that…. Like, on TV when they like, it's a dark room and like there's the criminal fella and then the police officer and the police officer is like … scary.[m]

For this person and many others, their only exposure to 'counselling' was through popular media which often reproduces stereotyped ideas of 'patients' lying on couches experiencing old fashioned psychoanalysis, or doctors and nurses forcibly medicating unruly psychiatric patients. One young person, unsurprisingly, had pictured the mental health service being located in something like an outdated asylum:

> Oh yes, I thought it would be like, like one of those mental hospitals, like the prisoners live there.[m]

The young people who took part in this study had been pleased to discover that their worst imaginings were not borne out in reality and that, for the most part, the mental health service they used was not as frightening and intimidating as they had anticipated.

When we asked young people about what would help them feel more able to use counselling services, they confirmed they would like more information about what the service would actually look like before taking the first step towards professional help. One of the things they thought would be helpful to them would be to see online images on the reception area of the clinic or the room in which the counselling took place. They also wanted to see pictures of the counsellors they might be speaking to. One young person explained how the combination of the unfamiliarity of the counselling environment and her exposure to popular media representations contributed to anxieties about seeing a counsellor for the first time:

> For me it's a very non-ordinary experience so I'm not sure what the expected 'etiquette' or something is. Basically, knowing what face-to-face counselling is actually like. My mind can't help but think of scenes from movies and TV for example since I know so little about counselling in general.[d]

There are also other ways that young people can be prepared for their first encounter with a mental health service. For example, in one of the services where we interviewed young Māori clients, they had used a cultural advisor to visit the young people and their families in their own homes, prior to their first session to explain how the service operated.[m] This had been very reassuring for the young people who were provided with this support and they told us how they appreciated this way of bridging their first encounter with the clinic. But this sort of mediated exposure to the counselling service seemed, from our interviews, to be the exception rather than the rule.

While most counselling spaces are usually not anywhere near as bad as some young people might imagine them to be, their position and design still do not always match with young people's preferences. Policymakers often emphasise the value of connecting medical health services with mental health services in keeping with notions of holistic health or in an attempt to position mental health as being similar to physical health. But there can be problems with locating youth counselling services within a physical health setting. A hospital or clinic building inhabited by doctors and nurses in uniform are a poor fit for young people looking for informal relationships and a relaxed, non-clinical atmosphere. As young people do not readily understand distress as a 'health issue' and instead see it as a more normalised response to life's difficulties, a medical environment seems particularly inappropriate. The young people we interviewed spoke about how they thought it would be better to integrate counselling services with youth clubs or other gathering places, and to use designs that ally mental health with social contact and recreational activity rather than with physical health interventions. They wanted these services to be close by in settings where they were already spending time. As one young person put it:

> It needs to be somewhere a lot of teenagers go, so it's like natural for them to go there.[o]

But it is not enough to simply move counselling spaces for young people away from medical settings. Young people also react to the way space is organised. One of the first experiences a young person will have of a counselling setting is the waiting area. One young client commented on how the layout and furnishings of the waiting room at the mental health service helped her to feel more comfortable:

> Yeah I thought it might be a bit different because they seemed like a family orientated place because they offer, I don't know, I felt like they offer a lot more … It isn't as serious as other places might be. Like you go in and there's just magazines everywhere and there's children's toys and there's a TV with children's videos and stuff … Yeah it was good to go into an environment where I felt comfortable.[1]

While in this example the young client clearly felt more at ease surrounded by children's toys as is common in child and adolescent mental health services, other young people might easily feel patronised and insulted by an environment so clearly set up for younger children. This can be a challenge when services for youth and children are being provided in the same setting.

Some counselling services are offered privately, in theory allowing counsellors more options to think about the preferences of their clients in the arrangements and décor of the space. By and large, however, the design of private practices seems often aimed rather more at impressing the parents rather than the young person themselves. One of the young people we spoke to talked about how he had been put off by the smooth, sophistication of the private consulting rooms where he saw a mental health professisonal:

> The first place I went to was … really formal. I felt kind of strange being there, I felt really uncomfortable, and it just wasn't really nice and it was a really sort of high class place and it was really expensive, and I was like I don't understand why it's so expensive and there were like weird candles and ornaments and things. It was really out of my comfort zone.[1]

Young people were able to give us a good sense of the building designs and décor they preferred. Most of them mentioned the need for informality and youth-friendly furnishings. One young person described her vision of a welcoming space, highlighting the contrast between this and the way that mental health services were usually arranged:

> I don't want to say like make it look like a kindergarten, but you know like make it a really happy place to be with lots of colours and stuff. Because a lot of the places you go they literally look like a hospital room or like a business office and you always think of the scenes in like movies where they're lying down on the couch with the clipboard and that's really not inviting.[o]

In workshops in which we asked young people to design their ideal services,[o] they substituted soft couches and beanbags for upright chairs. Ornaments and magazines in the waiting room were replaced with a table tennis table, books, and computer stations. Young people also offered a range of other creative suggestions for making the space more welcoming to youth such as including slides and games rooms, kitchens for making food, and quiet spaces where they could find privacy. While young people spoke about how counselling spaces could be made more attractive and fun for young people, the strongest sense we got from our interviews was that they were looking for an environment that would help them feel less nervous in this potentially intimidating encounter.

We spoke to young people at a school where the counsellors had obviously recognised the importance of a comfortable waiting space for young people. One young woman told us how, sometimes when she felt distressed, she would just go and sit in the waiting room without needing to see a counsellor. She explained how she and her friends took comfort simply from being outside of their classroom and in a space where they felt they could allow themselves to feel vulnerable:

> I think the times that I've left feeling better have been the times I've just sat and cried on the seat [in the waiting area], and I've just sat and cried and they've just left me there for the period and I sat and cried, and those are the times I've felt the best.[n]

Beyond the waiting rooms and broader environment, the design of the rooms in which the counselling takes place is also important. Most counsellors would be aware that sitting behind a desk in their counselling room would be inhibiting for young people. But beyond avoiding these obvious trappings of authority, there are some other ways that counsellors can make their rooms more conducive to young people. In my clinical work with teenagers, I found it helpful to have some objects, which could be idly toyed with, placed strategically around the room. Some magnets or a hacky sack have proved useful with a 14-year-old boy who might feel uncomfortable sitting still in a chair facing an adult. A low-key activity can provide a helpful distraction and take some of the pressure off 'having to talk.' Other young people like to supplement talking with art, making objects out of clay or drawing. The presence of these media in the room, even if they are not used, can help young people to feel like there is space for them to express themselves in whatever way they prefer. One popular counsellor at a local school had a room that felt comfortable and a set-up that enabled him to play music. One of his clients explained how these aspects helped her to feel more at ease in her initial counselling sessions:

> Like all the pictures and he seems to relate to kids like he just gets them to draw everything and he's got boxes of toys so kids can play with them if they want, plays their own music… I listen to music and that, just sat there and listen to music and it kind of calms it down.[n]

This same counsellor, apparently, would allow his young clients to construct their own playlists and played these when they returned for sessions, adding to the sense that this was their own space that could accommodate them as an individual and that they could use as they liked.

Young people also told us that they needed the counselling room to be a soothing space that allowed them to leave the pressures of the world behind them. One young woman explained how she saw the school counselling rooms as a place where she could escape from the difficulties she was experiencing in the classroom and school grounds:

> I was going through a hard time and I was feeling really upset. I wouldn't want to be sitting in class and being around people … So it was kind of like a refuge. You could go and get a bit of sanctuary somewhere.[n]

Another young person gave this description of an environment she would experience as peaceful and relaxing:

> I was thinking like a tranquil environment. So, to me that would be like water fountain thingies and like really calm, like nice music. So like, something that's really just relaxing so you can just really exist in the moment.[o]

In recent times, some mental health services have been more active in looking at how counselling spaces can provide specifically designed soothing environments for young people who are extremely distressed. Some services are providing 'chill rooms' where young people can sit by themselves, or with others, and settle their emotions. Acute mental health services have also started to offer specific 'sensory modulation' spaces where young people recovering from experiencing extreme distress can find comfort in a dimly lit room with soft furniture, weighted blankets, yoga mats, books, music and other calming sounds, sights, and smells.[117]

In addition to the counselling space needing to be relaxed, youth-friendly, and soothing, young people also told us of the significance of it feeling safe and, very importantly, private. With fears around confidentiality being so central for young people, it was unsurprising that those we spoke to were very conscious of the potential to be overheard through thin walls.[114] One young person described how she had noticed this:

> Something I would complain about is these walls you can hear everything through them, well I think you kind of can and so if someone is waiting in the waiting room and I'm talking. "Oh can they hear me?" because I can kind of hear sometimes when other people are in there if I'm in the waiting room.[o]

Young people also seemed highly aware of where the counselling services were positioned and what this meant for other people being able to see them come in for a session or leave. This was particularly an issue in relation to school counselling where, if the counselling service is located close to the classrooms or other social areas, it was very easy for other students to see a young person entering or leaving the building. Some of the better arrangements we came across in our research were when the counselling rooms were positioned inside a building behind the staff areas, making it less clear whether a young person was using the counselling service or seeing another staff member for a different reason.

But while the focus of this discussion has been on buildings and rooms, we also heard from young people about how they enjoyed opportunities to talk with counsellors outside of the confines of a building. Traditionally, counsellors have been concerned about maintaining their professionalism through the use of a dedicated 'working' space that helps them manage the boundaries of their relationship with their clients.[118] But young people do not seem to share these priorities, and they spoke about how they sometimes felt more comfortable talking in non-counselling spaces. It seemed that some of the services had recognised the greater ease of talking to young people outside of a consulting room, and we heard stories from some of the clients we interviewed about how they had appreciated an opportunity to speak to a counsellor more informally as they walked around the grounds of the service or were taken out to get some food at a local café. One young woman who had been seen at a hospital-based mental health service and had not been fortunate enough to have this experience captured the therapeutic benefits of holding a counselling session outdoors:

> Maybe they could take you out to somewhere like more, like representing New Zealand, like the bush and nature. The scenery that we have in New Zealand is real beautiful. Like maybe taking the kids out there and stuff and seeing the world, like appreciating the world and maybe having a picnic outside.[m]

For some young people, and perhaps particularly for young Māori and Pacific Islanders, it can also be appropriate to have counselling sessions in their home environment, and a few of the young people we spoke to had appreciated having someone come to their house to talk to them.[m] While this may be more culturally suitable for particular groups of clients, it can feed some of the anxieties that other young people have about their privacy and parents' involvement. A small number of young people also felt that having a mental health clinician visit them at their school was also helpful:

> Dealing with that is a lot easier now that I have help, and before to talk to them, like whenever, I can send her an email, and she makes it easier coming to my school as well. She comes and visits me at my school. It makes it a lot easier.[l]

The spaces in which young people get to speak to a counsellor matters to them. These spaces can signal formality, coldness, and authority or they can help young clients feel comfortable, soothed, and safe.

Getting access: *Getting in is a mission*

The main responsibility for the very low rates of mental health service use among youth can all too easily be put on young people themselves, to their own reluctance to surrender their agency, their lack of 'mental health literacy,' or their fear of stigma.[119] But it is important to highlight that many of the barriers that prevent young people from using professional support are not of their making. Even if young people finally take the difficult decision to seek help, they can face insurmountable difficulties in accessing it. One of the primary issues is the daunting logistics involved in finding their way to a place where they might get help. As I described earlier, many young people prefer to access services without their parents' involvement. However, it can be very difficult for a young person to organise a counselling session, outside of school or university setting, without having their parents involved. Unlike adults who can choose a counsellor online and call them to make an appointment, young people are often forced to negotiate a more complicated process that relies on the helpfulness of adults around them. Usually, young people need a referral from a teacher or general practitioner before they are seen by a mental health service, and this almost always involves their parents, at least for those who are below the age of consent (in New Zealand, this is not fixed but in reality tends to apply to young people below the age of 16).

Slightly older youth may be more able to access a service independently but doing so requires knowledge and skills. The young person would need to know how to contact the service and think through what they might need to say to get an appointment. While this can seem like an unproblematic process to professionals, for young people who have not previously done this, the challenges can be overwhelming. In discussions with young people, we found that one of the first barriers that they faced in seeking help with a mental health service included difficulties in finding basic information about what services might be available to them. Much of this information is available online but seldom presented in a coherent package and quite likely to be difficult to track down, especially if a young person is feeling emotionally overwhelmed at the time. One young person, we interviewed via instant messenger captured the difficulty of contemplating doing this alone:

> i literally wouldn't know where to start with finding a therapist, like i don't know if there's government ones or if you need private therapists. also the cost of it, i assume it would be expensive.[d]

When we spoke to young people we were also told about young people's lack of familiarity with making formal phone calls. When making an appointment by phone, they may not only be unsure about what to ask for or how to describe their circumstances but also, for a generation more at home with text than talk, a phone conversation with an unknown adult can be an intimidating task.

The logistics of organising transport to a service can also be daunting for a young person in distress. This might require, for example, planning a complicated bus route to arrive on time at an unknown destination, a demand that most adults might find taxing during a period of emotional turmoil. In addition, young people often do not have the freedom to organise their time as they wish. Even supposing they could access a free counselling service near to their home, they might still have to account to their parents for the time spent, possibly having to resort to deception to explain their absence over several hours during an afternoon.

There are also obvious cost barriers for young people in accessing mental health services although research suggests that, for teenagers, their parents may be more aware of this barrier than they are.[120] Some services are free, but these can be over-subscribed, require too much adult involvement, or be unable to provide the level or kind of support needed. In these situations, some young people would no doubt prefer private counselling services which may offer a more timely or tailored service. But the cost of these is often well beyond the reach of young people and the thought of requesting help from a parent might be too compromising, even assuming that their families could afford this expense.

Counselling based onsite at schools and universities helps to overcome some of these access challenges for those young people who are within these institutions. But despite the advantages of having access to free services nearby, some young people told us that they were worried about using these onsite services, stating concerns about the potential for breaches of confidence by the counsellor or the risk of being observed by peers. While these services remain an important resource for young people, for those not able, or unwilling, to use these, access to support may be difficult.

Beyond these barriers, one of the most significant difficulties that young people face in accessing counselling services are the very long waiting lists that mean that they are simply unable to see a professional in their time of need.[121] Young people who are reliant on the state mental health services for support with significant mental health problems seemed particularly aware of this problem. One of the young people we spoke to about barriers to accessing mental health services provided this tragic example:

> Yes there's some organisations I suppose and agencies. Sometimes getting into them is a mission in itself though. One of our friends actually this year was on the wait list to see mental health specialists but the wait list was so long she never got to see them and ended up taking her life actually.[d]

Other young people told us about their own painful experiences of being left waiting to be seen for longer than they could manage.

> They kept telling me there was a huge waiting list, which is really difficult to hear 'cause you're like, "What do I do in the meantime?" … I felt like they didn't really take me very seriously and I needed to do something really drastic to get up the waiting list.[k]

In another example, a young person who had struggled with a serious mental health problem spoke about how she felt she would not be seen unless she was a serious risk to herself and others:

> I called the Mental Health Line, just talked to them and then they couldn't do anything. They didn't actually do anything at all. The only way they would help me was if I say, "I'm going to kill this person. I'm going to hurt myself." There's really never any support for anyone unless they go to ED or something like that.[k]

The idea that young people in distress might need to wait until they are this desperate before they receive help has been borne out in discussions with my colleagues in the mental health services and in the recent government report on mental health services in New Zealand.[122] These observations paint a disturbing picture of a system in which clients are forced to wait until they are suicidal to be able to warrant being seen by a professional in the mental health system, where they are seen for just long enough to ensure their immediate safety. They are then discharged, only to return when they are once again in crisis. Even for milder problems, school and university counselling services run long waiting lists that may leave a young person in distress waiting weeks for an appointment. Many services also limit the number of sessions they will provide and these decisions are often based rather more on cost considerations than on the needs of an individual client.

Besides the distress entailed in not being able to receive help when and if they need it, one young person captured how it felt to be treated as though one's distress did not matter:

> When people are in that headspace they need support and to know people care. When they have to wait it makes them feel like they aren't worthy.[k]

For young people, there are many barriers in the way of accessing services. These include the logistical challenges of affording support, being able to get to the service and the freedom to do this when they want to. One of the most concerning issues is the shortage of services for young people that mean that many who might be in need of support are not able to be seen at the time that they need help — or indeed, in time to keep them safe from harm.

When people are feeling distressed and want to reach out for help, it can be extremely difficult to be told that they must wait for an appointment to talk about it. This waiting is likely to be difficult for anyone in distress, not just a young person. But for young people who are less used to delayed gratification and more used to acting 'in the moment,' these kinds of barriers can seem unintelligible as well as frustrating.

Needing flexibility: *Like whenever you need it*

When we interviewed young people, we were struck by the way they experienced time differently from the way that I experienced it in my generation. When I was younger, we would make an arrangement to meet someone at the cinema on a Friday night at 8.00 pm. We would normally have set up this arrangement earlier in the week and if anyone had to cancel, this would have been done via a phone call in advance. But digital technology has enabled young people to manage their time differently, with arrangements being much more fluid than they were previously, and organised according to whatever their moment to moment preferences might be.[103]

I became increasingly aware of this difference in the way we understood appointments during the process of interviewing young people for our research. There were, for example, many occasions on which I would arrive at a young person's home or school at our agreed time to find they were not there. After texting the participants, I might be told that they were at the mall with some friends or a sports event, and could we change the arrangement to another day. I got into the habit of texting young people before I set off on a, sometimes long, trip to see them just to make certain that their understanding of our meeting arrangements was the same as mine.

Given the way that young people manage their time arrangements, it was understandable then that one of the young people we interviewed about their counselling experiences expressed their surprise at why someone would need to wait for an appointment scheduled for the following week to discuss a problem that was worrying them "now."[j] The idea of booking an appointment and waiting for it, or indeed, even waiting during the period between weekly sessions seems foreign to young people. Instead, they envisaged a service in which they could simply walk in off the street in their moment of distress and ask to see a counsellor.

But despite young people's preferences for greater flexibility, most mental health services continue to require appointments to be made in advance. One of the strongest arguments against allowing for more flexible appointments has been the concern that the demand for services will exceed resources. Interestingly, some recent research suggests that walk-in clinics may be more cost-effective than running waiting lists.[123]

The need for flexibility is also present in young people's expectations of the way the therapy is conducted. Young people told us how they wanted their counsellors to adjust their availability to make it easier for clients to time their sessions for when they needed these. For one young woman who was struggling with ongoing psychological difficulties, what had been most valuable for her was being able to see her counsellor at the start of each day. She explained that this sense that she could see her counsellor when she needed to provided her with ongoing comfort:

> Even now I still go in and say hi in the morning, I'll pop my head around, she knows I'm there so I'll talk to her for a little bit.[n]

In my training as a psychologist, and in the training of many other mental health professionals, holding a fixed session time and not going beyond this was seen as central to holding the 'therapeutic frame.'[118] In theory, this was designed to help the client experience counselling as a predictable and protected space, which sat a little outside of their normal lives. It also, of course, helped professionals manage the structure of their working days and control their workload. While these are legitimate issues, our interviews with young people suggested that, in contrast with this rigid frame, they appreciated counsellors who were willing to 'bend the rules' and offer more flexible options for connecting than the traditional 50-minute, once a week session.

It was important to young people to feel that their counsellor would be responsive if they needed more support. For young people who have struggled with a lack of consistent and reliable support from their family or community, it was particularly important to know that someone would be there for them when they needed it. We heard some positive stories from young people who had a counsellor who was willing to make themselves available outside of the regular session times:

> We had an appointment every week pretty much and then like she asked me if I am really down and I needed to go more I could call her up and make another appointment. I didn't really do it. Like it felt good that I had a choice to do it.[l]

Many like this young client valued being given the option for flexible contact although most did not actually have to use it. Digital communication technology also allowed counsellors to make themselves more available than they might have previously:

> I guess the first kind of time we met she said "here's my email address if you need it. If you are feeling down and you want to talk to someone she said it's my work email so I will only read it during the week." I know that if anything does happen that I can turn to someone now. She's always going to be there and she will understand and help me out. It's nice … I haven't emailed her, but I know it's always there.[l]

The young people we spoke to also told us that it was helpful when counsellors allowed them to have shorter or longer sessions as needed. One young person spoke about how it had helped her to just speak to her counsellor about a particular issue for a short time rather than have a whole session:

> So the counsellor I see at school, I just about see her, like I come in and have a quick talk to her just about every day. Just stop in and talk with her, say whatever is on my mind and just go again.[n]

Young people also appreciated it when their counsellor recognised the other demands on their lives and tried to fit around this. For some young people struggling with the pressures to succeed and to meet the expectations of people around them, this recognition that they had other priorities was important:

> Then [the counsellor] said, "you know, every week we'll sort out a time on a different day so it doesn't affect your school work."[l]

Young people also described how they would have liked to have been able to have less support when they were feeling stronger and more when they felt vulnerable. One young client of a school counselling service described how she had made heavy use of counselling sessions the previous year when she was struggling, but now she felt better she needed to go far less often:

> I think this year I've only been down about 10 times max but last year every day probably. Sometimes twice a day, sometimes there'd be a gap, I wouldn't come down [to counselling]. Last year was a very bad year for me.[n]

From the perspective of counsellors, clients are often expected to agree upfront to a certain length of therapy (usually somewhere between four and 16 sessions) and anything less than this seems to demonstrate a lack of commitment from the client and risk the failure of the intervention. But these arrangements seem to be a poor fit with young people whose developmental needs vacillate and whose social world is far more fluid and changing. It may be that a model in which young people can step in and out of therapy as they need to is more in line with what young people need today.

One of the major challenges in making onsite support accessible to young people can be found in the clash between the carefully ordered and predictable systems valued by professionals and the flexibility which marks young people's social interactions. It would be important to differentiate between those aspects which enable the smooth functioning of services and those which are simply a result of convention and reluctance to change in order to better match young people's priorities for flexible access to counselling support.

Service providers and policymakers have been aware of the importance of young people being able to access support at the moment they need it. Telephone crisis lines have been operating for many decades now to provide counselling services that can be used anonymously during a period of crisis.[124] More recently mobile phone text (or online chat) counselling services have also been developed to allow young people to communicate with someone during a period of intense distress.[125] Young people talked about how, with these modes of counselling, they were freed from the challenges of finding their way to a counselling service and were able to make use of it where they were and when they needed it. We heard about how young people had made use of text counselling while at their desks in the classroom, from under their duvet at night and even while they sat in the bathroom at a party.

This mode of communication offers young people the opportunity to talk about problems with a counsellor at the very moment they are dealing with a difficult situation. One young woman, for example, told us how she texted a counsellor throughout a bus trip to school during which she was being bullied by other passengers. Another young man explained how he had been able to get text counselling support as he watched an escalating drunken conflict between family members who were in the kitchen with him at the time. Yet another young woman gave a poignant account of how important it had been for her to be able to text a counsellor for two days in which she was terrified she might be pregnant and until she got a negative test result:

> When I first told them, they went "Wow you must be going through a hard time because you don't have anyone to talk to." And you know I think I stopped texting them. And then later I texted them that I was at the doctor and the doctor said to me "Oh well, do you want me to do a blood test, be 100%?" I got him to do the blood test and everything and then yeah I texted the counsellor and they said "that's really great."[j]

The idea of being able to access this kind of immediate and ongoing support seemed to be a good fit for young people. One young person explained why she preferred this aspect of text counselling to scheduled face-to-face arrangements:

> [Text counselling] is not like every so often, it's just like whenever you need it.[j]

In this same study, participants spoke about how they valued that they had been able to stay in touch with the counsellor for as long as they needed, with the text counselling sessions lasting, in some cases, for a number of days:

> I thought they probably won't reply much. But they kept coming back and replying and I thought they would give up on me because I was a hopeless case, but they just kept coming back with ideas of how to cope with it, how to deal with it, ideas to approach my parents about how I am feeling.[j]

In contrast to those who appreciated being able to sustain a connection to a counsellor using text, others spoke about how they valued being able to stop the interaction when they no longer needed it. Whereas in face-to-face counselling sessions, a young person might be expected by convention or by the requirement to remain for the full hour's session regardless of how they were feeling, in text counselling young people can simply end the session when they feel better. One young client of the text counselling service captured this freedom:

> When I get real angry I take my phone and start texting, and then when they reply I am like: 'Oh I don't feel angry anymore.'[j]

But even while text counselling seems capable of meeting young people's need for immediate and flexible access, for some young people even a small wait between their message and a response from the counsellor was felt to be too much. One young person we spoke to clearly articulated her expectation of an immediate response:

> There is quite a break in-between when you text and when they text and you text back, that for me it didn't really work, that I would be waiting for a reply and I kind of expect things immediately and that doesn't always happen.[j]

It was clear from our research that digital services suffered from the same lack of resourcing as many of the face-to-face support services that young people might use. One of the biggest challenges is to make these services available 24 hours so that young people can access them during the night, which can be the time that they feel most alone and distressed. When we interviewed young people about when they had used the text counselling service, most of them spoke about making contact during the night as one young woman explained:

> I had a friend that died and yeah it was really messy and you know finishing school, that sort of thing so it would affect me most at night time when I was in bed and so I would just text Youthline so that I had someone to talk to mainly. Yeah all my other friends would sort of be asleep by that time. Yeah probably about like 10.30 or 11. It was quite annoying because they sort of stopped texting around midnight I think it is.[j]

For young people, it is difficult to imagine delaying access to support beyond the moment in which they are feeling intense distress as one of the text counselling clients described:

> I think I was like counting on it or something and it was night-time and they were like "Sorry we've got to go now." They asked, if you want to be texted back in the morning. But by the time of the morning it was already fine.[j]

In spite of the fact that text counselling and other digital services are not always available 24 hours a day, they have made access to counselling much easier for young people. In one of our studies, we analysed the transcripts of young people who had used the Youthline text counselling services during an episode of intense suicidality. Young people who contacted the service articulated the value of being able to reach out to someone via text in their moment of crisis, sometimes as they were about to attempt suicide. One young person, for example, texted that they were sitting on the edge of a building about to jump off.[p] The potential that digital technology has to offer young people support is considered further in Chapter 8.

It would be impossible to meet the needs of young people in distress without thinking carefully about the barriers to access. These barriers are substantial and include more than the practical inaccessibility of services. The notion of access needs to be broadened to include an understanding of young people's need to feel comfortable and welcomed into services as well as matching their new priorities for more flexible and immediate support.

What do young people want?

Young people want counselling and other support services that they can access easily and that fit around their own priorities. They want services that help them to overcome the many logistical barriers that get in the way of their finding help, and they need to have access to support that feels welcoming, unintimidating, and soothing.

Those working with young people can help them by

- Ensuring the availability of free or reasonably priced services that are located in areas that can be accessed without adult involvement.
- Designing counselling services that are attractive, informal, safe, and private.
- Exploring how counselling support can be made more flexible to fit around young people's changing needs.
- Advocating for more services so that young people do not have to manage long waiting times.
- Recognising the potential for digital resources to reach young people more immediately and in the spaces they inhabit.

8 Digital technology and mental health: *Chill and shoot zombies*

With an awareness that young people are high users of digital technology, mental health professionals and services have been quick to spot the potential to use this medium to reach those who might not be comfortable engaging face-to-face with a mental health professional.[126] In recent years, there has been a rapid proliferation of intervention options including online therapy and an ever-increasing number of apps designed to support young people with distress. It seems intuitively appropriate that given young people are using digital technology, the way to reach them is via this technology. However, professionals who have been working in this area have begun to understand that just 'going online' is not enough to connect with young people and that too often their well-intentioned efforts to design online interventions for this digital generation fall wide of the mark.

Adults have been described as 'digital immigrants' in comparison to youth who are called 'digital natives.'[127] While some adults object to the idea they may be less familiar with digital communication than young people,[128] it is difficult for them to fully fathom the way these technologies are deeply interwoven into the lives of a generation for whom it has shaped everything from their social relationships to their learning and leisure for as long as they can remember.

It has also been difficult for adults to keep up with the development of new social media platforms and the rapid shifts in fashions of use among young people. We have, for example, seen a mass migration of young people away from Facebook just as older people began to find a comfortable home there. Young people roll their eyes at Twitter and instead are more likely to use the image-based sites of Instagram, Snapchat, and YouTube to communicate with their peers.[129] TikTok is seeing a massive rise in popularity among youth as I write this,[130] but I have no doubt that it will be replaced by something else in the very near future. The eye-watering rapidity with which these platforms rise and fall in youth cultures leave those not immersed in the medium lagging behind in terms of their knowledge and understanding of young people's practices. I have had experiences of talking to young people in their late teens who laugh at their youthful commitment to Tumblr and confess wryly that they cannot keep pace with the changing preferences of their younger brothers and sisters. It is likely that we will soon have a cohort saying the same thing about TikTok. If young

DOI: 10.4324/9780429322457-8

people are struggling to keep up with new social media, the challenge would be far greater for those separated by a generation from young teens.

The difficulty that adults have in understanding how young people are using the internet may not just be due to their lack of familiarity with newer social media platforms. Adults and professionals are further disadvantaged in their knowledge of young people's online lives by being deliberately excluded from these. In our discussions with young people, we were told how some of their practices, such as having multiple accounts, are deliberately designed to ensure that their parents and other adults do not intrude into their private online interactions. While some adults believe that they know all about how their teenage children are using the internet, our discussions with young people suggest that this may seldom be the case.

Given the gap in knowledge and practice between youth and adults' online engagements, it is little wonder that interventions engineered by adults are not always greeted enthusiastically and embraced by this digital generation. If we are to find ways of connecting with young people online, we need to understand better how they negotiate their digital world and, more specifically, what it is that might help to engage them with mental health support in an online environment.

Finding safe digital spaces: *Do not talk to strangers on the internet*

It is ironic that while mental health professionals have rushed to explore the potential of the internet to host services that can support young people in distress, the blame for many youth mental health problems has been firmly attributed to this same medium. Much of the public discourse on digital technology has focused on the negative impacts it has had on young people's mental health.[131] Examples of online bullying have hit the headlines with stories of young people driven to suicide by merciless taunting on social media. There are disturbing accounts of grooming and sexual abuse through the internet as well as stories of young people sharing compromising photos of one another online. Access to pornography is also being recognised as a major problem for young people who are being shown that men being violent to women during sex is normal and expected.[132] These kinds of issues have been taken up by researchers who are rightly concerned about the impact these experiences have had on young people's mental health, and there is now a wealth of data that highlights the risks of being exposed to abusive material or being bullied and abused online.

Research suggests that many young people have been bullied online.[133] The young people we spoke to did acknowledge online bullying as a source of difficulty for today's youth, and occasionally, we were told stories of young people who had been subjected to difficult experiences on social media such as the example below given by a young man who was concerned about his younger sister:

> Yeah so my sister has struggled with depression and anxiety since she started high school. This tended to centre around relationships with friends.

> She would often rant about the two-faced nature of people when interacting via social media - that they can be pleasant in person, but horrible online. She would frequently get very upset.[i]

But on the whole, we heard surprisingly few accounts of either experienced or witnessed online bullying. This may be because most of the young people we spoke to were a little older and cyberbullying is thought to be more common for younger adolescents.[134] But some young people also seemed to think that while cyberbullying existed, it was not the only, or even the most significant, issue for many young people. As one of the school students we spoke to put it:

> Yeah, there's one instance of cyberbullying and it gets blown up on the media like it's this huge problem and it's happening everywhere... Yeah, there have been cases for like one or two people, not for like masses.[b]

Our interviews with young people suggested that, for them, the internet is not seen as the primary source of their problems but rather just a vehicle through which the challenges they faced in their real lives were expressed. As one young woman explained:

> There's the danger of getting support from the wrong person like if they add someone they don't know on social media and that person tries to help in a dodgy way. But yeah, I wouldn't recommend getting advice from people you dont know in real life either. Also there is the risk of bullying if they are at high school or school or anywhere really...at school or social functions like parties.[i]

Young people also seem to have a more nuanced understanding of the potentials of social media for both abuse and support. Ironically, given the association of the internet with bullying, we were given several examples of how online support had actually helped to counteract the bullying that young people experienced in real life. As one young woman explained:

> Its kinda like how in school when kids would get bullied they were always told in anti bullying assemblies to tell an adult or a teacher. People didn't like that option so they just never reached out. I think if more people were aware of safe spaces on the internet they could benefit because certain people wouldn't want to 'risk' saying something irl and occasionally talking about stuff online can give people the courage to talk about stuff outside of the internet.[i]

Another young boy told a poignant story of how he was being mercilessly bullied at school and when an older boy asked him how he was in a private message on Facebook, he finally found the courage to tell him what was happening. The next day the older boy met him at the school gates to walk him to school and continued to do this until the bullying had stopped.[i]

Furthermore, rather than focusing on extreme cases of online bullying and abuse, the young people we spoke to often seemed more concerned with the 'everyday' challenges they had to negotiate in the online world. For example, they paid more attention to the pressure of maintaining a positive online identity, the seduction of appearing 'popular,' the temptation to compare themselves to others, and concern about privacy issues.

In many ways, the anxieties young people held about online behaviour were not dissimilar to those they worried about in real life. Nonetheless, the way that these pressures were reflected in visible forms on social media was recognised to be particularly difficult for young people. Even those young people who were strongly invested in using social media seemed to be aware of the risk of getting too caught up in needing to be liked and comparing the quality of their lives to those of their friends, as one young person who we interviewed as part of our digital mental health study explained:

> so, i've realised i've been so attached to my phone recently and wasting time looking at other people's lives through what they post on snapchat and Instagram. For example in the holidays i felt it made me feel kinda left out when im seeing posts of people doing things, when i'm not even that close with them and i realised it's kinda affecting me more than i thought...[q]

This comment also raises the question of 'internet addiction' which is one of the concerns that are most frequently raised by adults in relation to youth mental health.[135] This label, which draws from the concept of physical addiction to a substance, is meant to capture the potential for young people to become dependent on the cheap thrill of a 'like' on their social media post or the adrenalin rush of gaming to the exclusion of their offline lives. While the notion of a gaming addiction was considered as a potential diagnostic category in the most recent edition of the DSM-5, the analogy with chemical addiction is perhaps a little bit of a stretch. The overuse of the internet lacks some of the biological features associated with addiction and may be more likely to be an expression of other mental health difficulties.[136] Interestingly, the focus on the object of addiction is also perhaps out of step with new thinking in the addiction area that this behaviour has less to do with biology and more to do with other lacks in people's lives, particularly the absence of meaningful relationships.[137] Loneliness, for example, has been found to contribute to young people's reliance on the internet.[138] The latter way of thinking about the overuse of gaming or other activities on the internet may draw attention back to some of the more general issues that young people struggle with such as social isolation or other pressures from which gaming might be a respite.

Nonetheless, the young people we spoke to did seem wary of the potential to overuse digital technology. Although most of those we interviewed as part of our research on digital mental health were comfortable about being high users of social media, we did occasionally hear from young people who had become concerned about how much time they were spending online. We spoke to a few young people who said they were deliberately making the choice to move away from social media because of its negative impact on their mental health. While this was a relatively small proportion of the young people we interviewed, the potential for a trend away from social media among young people has been noted in recent surveys.[139] Some disaffection with social media was particularly evident among some of the Māori and Pasifika young people we interviewed, who spoke about the dangers of losing the face-to-face connections which were so important in their cultures. One young Māori man explained how he felt technology placed barrier in the path of establishing real connections with people:

> Yeah. I think even like, *kanohi ki te kanohi* or face to face, um, it can be hard to develop a relationship and to feel like someone genuinely cares about you through a device. And because we associate mobile phones with a level of detachment, even technology is quite detached you know?[q]

But this same young man went on to talk about how difficult it was to give up on social media altogether explaining, paradoxically, that this would mean giving up on an important source of social connection:

> And then, there's a layer of disconnect. Because suddenly like you feel quite um, "Oh if I delete... my Facebook, I won't be able to keep up with the cuzzies in Australia kind of thing". You know, are they going to call me? Probably not. But will they post on Facebook ten times a day? Yeah, probably. And you kind of miss out. You feel like you're missing out on certain milestones, you know... you retain your social media applications for that, for that reason.[q]

This ambivalence about social media was not unusual, and some young people who said they wanted social media to play less of a role in their lives were still apparently using a variety of platforms to mediate various activities. The small group of young people who were concerned about their generation's overuse of social media, for example, still mentioned using YouTube for entertainment, Reddit for information, Spotify to listen to and share music playlists, and Discord to game with friends. One young woman who told us she was in the process of giving up social media, gave us a sense of how important digital connection remained in her life:

> Um, my phone, probably not so beneficial. But my laptop, very beneficial because... uni. I guess, and it also depends. Like, my timetable app, I look at it all the time. I find it so helpful, and it's on my phone. Um, and I mean, Snapchat is my primary use that I contact my friends. Like, 'are you going to a lecture', or something, so, I guess that is beneficial. Um, but scrolling through Instagram and Facebook isn't.[q]

It seems that for young people in this generation, digital communication is so deeply integrated into their lives that they hardly register its existence. This is reminiscent of the famous quote from the media critic, Marshall MCluhan, that fish are the last to discover water.[140]

Young people have also been well-educated about the risk of exposing private information about themselves online and the implications that this might have for their future. Most of those we spoke to seemed very aware of the potential for online information to be able to be accessed by other people who could influence their future. For example, one young man explained how it would be important to be careful about what information he put out on social media about himself as it could affect his career:

> I think it does come with a kinda big risk because it can easily influence how others see you and if an employer looks see it can influence their decision to hire you as well.[i]

Beyond these dangers, young people also seemed particularly cautious about the potential for more corporate interests to invade their 'private' internet space. In many ways, they seemed far more alert to the influence of algorithms to advertise products or sinister bots to produce false content than older users of the internet, as though they had developed a sixth sense for what can be trusted. In general, young people seem to approach information from unknown sources with considerable healthy scepticism. The idea that social media users are being used by corporate interests was captured in the documentary *The Social Dilemma* where the primary message was: 'If you are not paying for the product; *you* are the product.'[141] This threat resonates strongly with young people who are particularly concerned with threats to their agency and privacy.

But while young people were aware of the risks of the internet and social media, they seemed to hold a more balanced view, recognising a tradeoff between the risks of online engagement and the advantages this also gave them. While adults often represent risks of the internet for young people as part of a dangerous new phenomenon, for young people the risks seemed to be understood as just another set of challenges they needed to learn to negotiate, not very different to the challenges they were also struggling within their offline worlds. Instead of seeing themselves as 'victims' of the internet, they positioned themselves as being able to make active choices about how to use it. Furthermore, rather than seeing social media as an insurmountable threat, they emphasised their own role in developing the skills to maximise its benefits while minimising the dangers. For some young people, the solution to these challenges had been to abandon social media, but for the majority, it was a matter of negotiating their way through the risks and looking for interactions that were helpful and supportive. One young woman explained how she felt it was important for adults to help young people manage the risks of the internet rather than offering unhelpful generalisations about the dangers:

> It is really difficult because adults constantly tell teenagers "dont talk to strangers on the internet" but it can be really supportive environment ... I think instead of saying don't talk to strangers on the internet, young people should be given resources on how to find good support groups on social media, warning signs of a bad support group etc.[i]

While there are risks involved in digital communication and especially social media, the advice to 'get off your phone' may only serve to alienate this new generation who have a more nuanced understanding of the challenges of social media and awareness of its relationship with the broader challenges facing young people. Furthermore, to put the blame for young people's mental health problems purely on social media, falls into the trap of 'blaming the messenger' rather than recognising the legitimacy of the difficulties that young people face in the 'real world.' This was highlighted in a meme that has done the rounds on young people's social media recently that goes something like this: 'We don't have jobs or money and climate change is destroying the world. But parents be like: "Social media is making young people anxious".'

Using digital resources: *Is it worth engaging with?*

In spite of the concerns that mental health professionals seem to hold about the negative effects of the internet on young people's lives, an increasing number of researchers and service providers are exploring ways that online resources can be used to provide interventions aimed at supporting young people online.[142]

One of the ways that the internet is thought to be able to facilitate youth mental health is by providing information that helps young people to identify whether they have a problem like 'depression' or 'anxiety' and suggesting strategies and resources that might help them.[143] This is in line with broader efforts designed to improve the 'mental health literacy' of young people.[144] However, there are challenges in ensuring that young people get helpful and accurate information about mental health issues. One of the most well-recognised challenges in online information seeking is simply that there is so much material available that it is difficult for young people to know where to focus their attention.[145] When we interviewed young people about how they looked for information on mental health, they explained how this could often be overwhelming:

> In truth there is already a lot of info online. If I were to make the right searches I'd be bombarded with all of this info which would supposedly help me... For first time info getters, it may seem a bit overwhelming, and prevent us from going back.[d]

The internet is also host to information which is inaccurate and unhelpful in the area of mental health.[146] Some of the misinformation on mental health problems may arise from the well-intentioned ignorance of the posters but might also sometimes be a function of more sinister motives to provide 'malinformation' from people who have serious mental health problems themselves or problematic political agendas. There may also be risks that arise from inaccuracies in direct to consumer advertising for psychiatric medications like antidepressants.[147] The young people we spoke to seemed very aware of the potential to be deliberately misled by mental health information on the internet. As one young woman put it:

> i think be careful who you take advice from, there're lots of people online who say if you buy their product / plan / whatever it'll fix all your problems and sometimes it's hard to know who you can trust.[d]

While the risks of false information on the internet are well-recognised, there can also be negative outcomes that go unrecognised from young people engaging even with accurate mental health resources. In one of our studies, we came across a group of high school students who had been referred by a teacher to a, no doubt reputable, mental health site where they could complete an online quiz to check whether they suffered from depression. When we spoke to some of those who had completed the online assessment, they seemed overall rather perplexed and unnerved by the experience. One young woman captured the discomfort of completing the quiz and being informed that she had 'mild depression.'

> Yeah, it really did. I was like 'do I?' I had to question myself like … because the answers I gave were honest so like I probably do and I answered everything right and then … yeah. I didn't really do anything about it though … Yeah, I looked at it and I was like … "I dunno?" I did it at home and I was looking at it and I was like 'do I want to know more or do I just want to ignore it' and I was like 'ignore it' so I completely ignored it. I think I was scared of knowing exactly what it was and how you get it and things like that.[q]

This young woman went on to tell us that she spoke to other students in her class who had also been told they had the same diagnosis, and the general consensus had been to disregard it. It was clear though that some of these young people had been left feeling worried about their own mental health and uncomfortable with the idea that they had something wrong with them.

Fortunately, most of the young people we spoke to seemed to be cautious about simply accepting information they read on the internet and rather than relying on Google searches for advice or information, most tended to look for support and recommendations from people who had an online presence they trusted. Some of these trusted people were media influencers who had made it part of their mission to educate and help young people with mental health problems — often revealing that they themselves had struggled with similar issues. One young person we interviewed about finding support online clarified the key elements that drew young people to certain media influencers and made them more inclined to follow their advice on mental health issues:

> because they're people similar to oneself talking about their relatable experiences so they also sound like a friend.[d]

A video format in which people could be seen and heard also seemed to give a greater sense of connection and intimacy with the person speaking. As one young person explained:

> This is because videos on YouTube makes the person feel he/she is sitting with the other one. They see and hear them. And plus they know that person is a real person.[d]

The young people we spoke to seemed willing to listen to advice from people who had a trusted and visible presence online but also particularly sought out those ideas that matched with their own values and opinions. The young people we spoke to explained how they tended to follow and 'listen to' personalities who shared a similar set of values or had experienced similar problems:

> I'm mainly on Instagram and I have lots of … influencers that I really like going to. I have strong feminists … So I like people like that who aren't scared to share that they are different and that being different is okay … I like to follow a lot of female how to do say it? Activists? They are just really empowering and strong and I like it.[q]

Young people did not seem to treat mental health knowledge as factual information based on science and those who provided this information were not generally seen as experts. Instead, the young people we spoke to often conveyed the idea that each person should weigh up the information available to see to what extent it might fit with who they were as an individual and what they needed. As one young person explained:

> Um, it has actually helped me a lot because like on Instagram, I follow like psychologists and stuff like that, and sometimes it's good in terms of like … unpacking certain like traumas or stuff like that. But … there needs to be some sort of understanding that it's just a very general and probably quite individual thing that they're doing or that they're sharing so it might not work for you or it might not be relevant to you. Like, not everything you read on the internet is like relevant to you, or true to you.[q]

In addition to mental health information online, there has been a proliferation of apps specifically designed for mental health as well as mental health interventions. Some of these have been carefully designed such as the CBT-based SPARX programme developed by colleagues in New Zealand.[148] But there are countless other apps available for young people to manage their mental health and not all of these have been designed with professional input. The lack of oversight of these resources has led the internet to be labelled the 'wild west' of mental health care.[149]

Among those young people we interviewed for our research, there were some who had used apps to manage their mental health, with probably the most commonly mentioned being those used to facilitate 'mindfulness.' Some young people were making good use of mindfulness resources to counter the pressures they experienced as one young Māori man described:

> I put on my headphones, and I just – usually I've had a pretty big day and you know, with exercise and study, and you know, just having good kai [food] and when you live like a decent life like that it's pretty easy to go to sleep and when you're living kind of full on I suppose but … yeah, I just usually meditate um, I listen to these files, I have on my phone. Then once I finish meditating then I just go to sleep while listening to the meditation files I have on my phone.[q]

More frequently though we were given a somewhat mixed picture of young people's willingness to engage with professionally designed resources online or via apps. One young man explained how he had become disillusioned with the process of setting up the apps and the charges associated with some of these:

> Nah, I don't really mess with a lot of apps. Um, too distracting and then fuck, you get caught up trying to set it all up. And like you're saying, you get charged for some of the decent apps you can get, they charge you, you know? It just pisses me off, aye.[q]

Another young person conveyed the sense that these professionally designed resources were perhaps not being used as widely as might be thought:

> I think there is a level of – is this effective? Like, is it worth like, engaging with? … I think there are more tools available to us. But as to whether or not we're utilising them, I don't think we are um, utilising them as much as the people who have developed them want us to.[q]

Overall, our interviews with young people suggested that, rather than relying on professionally designed tools, they had devised their own digitally enhanced strategies for dealing with emotional distress. One young woman, for example, spoke about how she had found more idiosyncratic ways of using digital resources to manage her mental health:

> I think what I usually end up doing is not using specific mental health apps but using apps that I know will kind of like calm me down if I'm using them. Like, have you ever played Boggle? Because I have this thing on my phone

> and you can like play Boggle with other people and I know that doing that calms me down. So it's kind of not specifically a mental health app but like a, an app that's being repurposed for mental health purposes if that makes sense...[q]

This idea of repurposing games or developing creative strategies using digital resources was a common theme in our interviews, and one young woman explained how she used the notes function on her phone to calm herself down when she needed to:

> Yeah, um, I actually do not have like a good definition of what an app is,, but I do have like a notes thing on my phone, I end up just typing out loads of like poetry and just like random thoughts and like a kind of half-baked political analysis that might be useful in something else, three weeks afterwards. And that kind of helps as well. Um, and then the thing that I use to record voice notes on my phone for like recording music and stuff that can be useful as well. So many the stuff that's already there just kind of, yeah, being repurposed.[q]

We also heard from young people about how they used online gaming and listened to music on Spotify to manage their distress or to change their mood.

Professionals who design mental health resources for young people may see themselves as offering ready-made tools or interventions to young people to help them with their mental health. Our conversations with young people suggested instead they were picking and choosing from digital technology to find those, largely informal, resources that they were able to tailor to meet their specific needs. As Ito and her colleagues put it, it might be more appropriate to think of young people on the internet as patrons at a buffet who can take what they need when they want rather than imagine them as passive recipients of professional interventions.[103]

Overall, the relationship that young people have with online support may be more complex than has been thought. It is not just a matter of designing interventions that are thought to be 'youth friendly' and delivering them through this medium. Instead, it is important to recognise that young people are active participants, finding, selecting, and repurposing online resources in ways that suit their own needs. As with their engagement with face-to-face support, the options offered to them need to respect their agency, their individuality, and their need for a trusting relational connection.

Finding support: *Texting is much more comfortable*

Interactive text counselling with a real person in real-time may have more potential than other professional online mental health resources to reach young people in distress.[150] As described in the previous chapter, this form of counselling enables young people to communicate with a counsellor via text (or online chat) and is increasingly been offered as an alternative to the more traditional telephone counselling lines which were intended to meet the immediate need of people in crisis. As with the crisis lines, the digital service is anonymous with neither the counsellor's nor the client's identity being revealed.

In New Zealand, Youthline began offering a small-scale text counselling service as an adjunct to their telephone and face-to-face service in 2004. The demand for this service rapidly eclipsed their other services as they began to receive hundreds of texts each day. We interviewed young people who had used this service to find out how they had experienced it and, in particular, how it compared to other forms of support they had available to them.

Mental health professionals who are less familiar with online communication have been sceptical about whether meaningful conversations can be conducted through the relatively short texts on which this form of counselling relies. Those young people who had used this service, however, told us they felt more comfortable talking in this medium than they did in face-to-face communication. One young client captured the contrast between the way she felt during text counselling and the discomfort she felt in talking face-to-face with an adult counsellor:

> I guess texting is much more comfortable because when they talk I can't look directly in their eye. I have to look everywhere in the room, which is quite awkward.[j]

It seemed that the young people also felt the benefits of what researchers have called the 'disinhibition effect,' produced by the distance and anonymity of this form of digital communication.[151] In general, the young people we spoke to said they found it easier to confide sensitive issues via text. It appeared that not being known to the counsellor freed them from the fear of judgement that would normally deter them from using a face-to-face service. The absence of auditory and visual cues indicating the counsellor's response also seemed to provide young people with a much-needed respite from dealing with other people's needs and expectations as one young woman explained:

> It's like cause I trust our school counselor, but at times it's just if like I thought that they would judge me cause she knows me and she knows what I was going through before, because my mum called the school and stuff. That's why sometimes I just text Youthline because I trust them more, because they don't really know me and I know that they won't judge me.[j]

The freedom that text counselling gave young people to talk about sensitive issues was borne out in their use of the service to talk about suicide. Young people who had texted in when feeling suicidal often commented that they would have only been able to tell someone through this medium. As one young client expressed to her counsellor:

> I won't ring if I was in serious trouble or in a harmful situation I would only be able to text.[p]

Another advantage of this service from the young clients' perspectives was being able to get support without having to reveal their difficulties to their parents. The young people we spoke to provided examples of how they had been able to text a counsellor privately from their bedrooms without their parents knowing and sometimes even from the sitting room with their parents and other adults close by. One young person captured how important this was to her as she was not normally allowed the freedom to make her own decisions about who she could talk to:

> Yeah. I kind of thought texting was a lot easier just because Mum and Dad were at home and I didn't want them, like [to hear] me talking on the phone [because] they would get curious as to who I was talking to. I didn't really want them to walk in and ask who I was talking to and I couldn't exactly say Youthline, because then they would be like oh what are you talking to Youthline for? So I kind of thought texting sort of was a bit safer.[j]

The opportunity to express themselves through text was seen as one of the most valuable aspects of this form of counselling. The young people we interviewed explained that this medium allowed them the space to work out what they wanted to say and sometimes also to reflect on, and make sense of, how they were feeling. Given the difficulties that young people experience in gathering their thoughts and putting their opinions across in the presence of an adult counsellor, this may be a particularly helpful aspect as this young woman explained:

> Like I find it easier in like writing stuff down. Yeah, I feel more secure. I don't know why, but it's just like cause you can see the words that you're writing… in text you have time to process everything so you can like think about what you are going to say, but in [face-to-face] counseling you have to think really fast.[j]

In listening to young people's accounts of how they communicated their innermost thoughts through text, I was reminded of a comment from an online researcher, James Alleman, that anyone who has written a love letter understands that it is possible to express ourselves meaningfully to people we cannot hear or see. As I discussed in Chapter 6, text counselling was also able to offer a surprising degree of relational connection for young people who were looking for this.

But in spite of hearing largely positive accounts of the way in which text counselling was able to meet young people's needs for connection, there were still some who told us that their preference was to connect face-to-face with a counsellor. One young man explained why he had chosen to cancel a counselling session which had been going to be offered online during the COVID-19 lockdown:

> I feel like, there are some things that sometimes when you're seeing, when you're with someone in person that you don't know you might – you kind of get the general mood. Like, how much do I think that I should share? Um, and, like there … yeah. So, I actually just cancelled the session when they told me they were only doing those two forms at the moment and I was like, oh I'll come back when you know, when it's back to like, the regular in-person stuff. Um, because, I might … you know sometimes you can kind of read the body language and like, 'oh actually maybe I would – this person is not so bad, maybe I can share more.'[q]

Even when young people are willing to engage with digital support, this may not be the most suitable option for all. Some young people simply seemed to prefer face-to-face support. In other cases, they were struggling with more significant issues and needed a higher level of support than a digital conversation could offer. Nonetheless, it is clear that text counselling provided a helpful way for some young people to talk about the things that mattered to them.

But just as they do in their offline lives, young people are far more likely to look for support from their friends and peer networks than from professionals or professional websites. This informal space in which young people might talk about mental health issues online is often depicted as being fraught with risk for young people. Some of the negative representations of the internet have emphasised the disturbing images that young people post of self-harm, including graphic images, apparently intended to elicit 'help' from their networks but often generating shock and discomfort among other young people.[152] Those we spoke to were aware of these kinds of posts and were mostly disturbed by their content. But while this might represent some of the social media posts on mental health, our discussions with young people revealed much more sensitive and gentle interactions between young people feeling distressed and others offering them support.

Giving and receiving support seemed to be a commonplace experience for young people in online contexts. However, there seemed to be general agreement that emotional safety was a prerequisite for being able to reach out to peers for help on the internet, just as it is in other areas of help-seeking. One young person we interviewed about peer support online succinctly summed this up in the phrase:

> It takes trust to talk about these issues.[i]

Young people were clearly more comfortable talking openly about their distress in 'friend groups' where safety seemed to be protected by a set of unspoken rules. Similarly, they spoke about only responding to signs of distress when they knew the person well, personally. In public domains, support was often expressed quite simply through a sympathetic emoji or comment but most young people seemed to recognise an imperative to shift the discussion quickly from the public into private online channels for more intimate conversations. These unspoken rules were articulated in the following account from a young person:

> I don't really supportively comment on people I don't know very well because it often doesn't feel like the right place. But if anyone I knew posted something distressing I would message them and ask them how they are.[i]

Although many of those we spoke to, only asked for or received support from people they knew in friendship networks, there were some who used online support forums. Even in these settings, safety remained a priority and young people were clear that they would only talk openly in forms where there was good moderation and clear rules for engagement, as one young woman explained:

> You want a group with 2+ admins so its monitored closely and comments that are reported getting taken down fast. And obviously read the group rules making sure there is focus on being respectful.[i]

Some participants also described how they felt safe in networks where they could communicate anonymously. Several participants referred specifically to Discord which is primarily intended for gaming but which young people are able to set up groups where they can also chat as they game. In these contexts, it seemed that it was not only the anonymity which provided the safety to share confidences but also that there was a growing sense of connection between users that enabled the development of trust over time:

> Certainly, maybe its the anonymity of Discord … And with that too I think talking to people about these issues you often can get really close really fast- because of the trust that it does take to talk about these issues, which could lead them to be far more honest about it.[i]

Our conversations with young people provided many examples of posts in which they had reached out for help from one another. One of the screenshots provided by a participant, for example, included a post that said:

> [name] is feeling dysphoric [sad emoji]. If anyone wants to send me messages of validation it would be much appreciated right now.[i]

But it was also intriguing to hear from young people that it was more common for them to express their distress obliquely, if at all. As one young woman we interviewed explained, distress was seldom conveyed directly and mostly young people 'just hint' at their distress. She went on to explain how a sense of shame often made it difficult for young people to express their distress directly, citing her own experience as an example:

> More or less because I was ashamed of being depressed but still needed the help but didn't quite know how to get the help as I did not want to ask directly at all.[i]

In keeping with this, many young people spoke about how they were attuned to picking up peers' indirect expressions of distress. In much the same way as someone might notice a friend looking a little down or being less sociable than usual, young people have learned to 'read between the lines' of online posts to recognise when a friend might need help. One young woman described the oblique messages she had learned to interpret in her online networks:

> so today a friend of mine posted on her third account saying "why is nothing making sense"… another example is someone posting a photo rolling their eyes but without a caption…[i]

Young people explained how they were on alert for subtle changes in their friends' online behaviour as an indication that they might need support. Another young woman described how she was able to identify people who might need help in this way:

> It's usually when people suddenly stop posting happy smiling pictures or place captions on their posts which aren't their usual selves that I ask how they are feeling…[i]

Another young woman explained how she had put together her friend's changed online behaviour with knowledge of some family problems she was having to aid her realisation that her friend might be struggling:

> Well yeah, because we had been talking all the time it seemed in the last few days and then she suddenly wasn't being as responsive and started giving shorter less detailed replies.[i]

Through our research on peer support online, we got in touch with a group of young people who clearly saw themselves as playing a significant role in noticing and responding to people's distress in various social media forums and groups. These young people's accounts demonstrated the careful way they went about assessing whether a friend might need help. For example, one young woman who spent a great deal of time helping others on social media talked about how she watched for dark humour which she believed revealed something of how people really felt. As she explained:

> Well for me I always assume any joke someone makes or funny suicide depression meme has some truth to it.[i]

In the same vein, another participant in this study described how she recognised aggressive posts as a cry for help:

> like when I was a kid and got hurt my parents coming over to hug me would only make me feel more upset and I'd lash out at them... so I think it's something that I personally recognise in others.[i]

Some young people seemed to have trained themselves to be particularly alert to signs that a person might be experiencing mental health problems as one participant put it:

> Well I mean I always watch for warning signs, depressed posting, distance from talking for a while.[i]

But even for those less obviously committed to 'helping' online, there was broad agreement that many young people were actively looking for, and receiving, support on social media.

While the popular conception of online support often involves receiving some sort of practical mental health advice, this seemed to be the least preferred option for young people. In fact, in a survey we conducted with 385 university students to find out about their online support practices, less than 15% identified practical advice as a as a helpful response. Most of the young people we spoke to were clear that the most important thing one young person could do for another was to simply listen. One young person who described themselves as 'gender non-conforming,' provided this detailed account of what it meant to 'listen' in an online environment:

> I will receive a huge block of text and may just reply with a "Yeah that sucks. Where to from now?" Or even interject between messages with a classic "yikes" or "oof" or even just a ":/"[i]

Beyond having someone listen to their problems, young people seemed to be looking for some sort of affirmation or encouragement from their online networks. We were given many examples of how young people might respond to distress with a phrase like: "You'll be ok. I know this is a tough patch but you will come out the other side of it stronger" or with heart or care emojis, or with emojis of sad or angry faces to demonstrate empathy. Young people who need support find it comforting to feel that someone cares about their struggles as one young woman explained:

> Responses checking in or asking how I am are helpful because it lets me know that people care. Sometimes people just remind me that they love me and that's probably the most helpful because if I'm worthy of their love I must be alright then.[i]

While the young people we spoke to seemed willing to respond to people who were distressed, they were also very sensitive about the potential for intrusion, being careful to adjust their responses to what the person needed:

> Yeah and sometimes they don't want to open up or say they're "fine" so I usually would take the conversation in a different direction because I don't want to make them uncomfortable or force them to talk.[i]

It seems that even young people who are keen to help others are aware of the potential for undermining the privacy and agency that their generation values. Their accounts often showed considerable sophistication in the way they were able to offer help in ways that were respectful of this need. One participant gave the following detailed account of the typical way she would manage a sensitive online conversation:

> I usually manage the conversation just by controlling the flow of it, which is a balance of expressing sympathy and understanding, and trying to move to whatever I need to ask next. With most people they either just say okay and shift the conversation to how I am and I let the conversation flow that way. But at the end let them know I am here for them if they want to talk or they just say they are not okay and I listen to then rant and offer to hang out or something to help with how they feel.[i]

In some cases, young people explained that support was best provided by just being there. One young man explained how he might respond to a friend who was going through a difficult time:

> It was as simple as playing an online game with them as it gave them company. They don't really like sharing but rather know someone is out there for them. Then we'd chill and shoot zombies or something. I'd poke to check if they would talk about it like "hey so I heard what happened..." And they'd usually respond with like "yeah I'm okay".[i]

But of course, not all expressions of distress are met with tactful or kind responses and young people who reveal their vulnerability might be subject to the same meanness and lack of care that can be found in other online and offline interactions.

In the university student survey I described earlier, we asked specifically about the negative responses that young people had witnessed in relation to expressions of distress on social media. In keeping with our other research studies, there seemed to be little focus on what might be considered overt instances of bullying or aggressive responses. Only a very small proportion (2%) of the young people who took part in our survey described seeing forms of abuse in which people are encouraged to "go ahead and kill themselves,"[g] a phenomenon which has perhaps received disproportionate attention in the popular media. Nonetheless, this study did suggest that other kinds of negative responses were common including those which minimised distress or made fun of the person who had shown their vulnerability. These kinds of responses typically included things like being told to "toughen up," or "get over it," or laughing emojis or acronyms like LOL (laughing out loud).[g]

It may be that because of these unkind responses that not all the young people we spoke to felt comfortable sharing their distress with others online. Some young people were rather more cautious about expressing their vulnerability in online contexts, citing the potential for even supportive networks to become unhelpful when young people got caught up in reinforcing one another's difficulties. One young woman described her increasingly negative experience of being part of an informal online support group:

> I was going on there for validation if I'm being I thought I was going on there to get better, but actually – and sometimes it becomes quite echo chamber-y, because you're all kind of sharing all of this stuff, and it can lead to further issues around like, what you're going through. It can like, lead to... yeah. Because suddenly all the people on there are, you know. Yeah. So, it becomes like a bubble. And, you're not really getting help, per se. You're just kind of getting people reinforcing those ideas. Yeah.[q]

In addition to the risks of amplifying young people's difficulties in online networks with peers, there is also the potential for these support networks to replace offline help-seeking rather than facilitate it.[153] Although this is possible, we also heard from some young people about the important role that online friends could play in encouraging them to seek support from an offline counsellor when they needed this. They spoke about how they would be more likely to approach a counsellor with individualised guidance from someone they trusted online as one young person articulated:

> So someone I trust in this way telling me they support me seeking out further help, or maybe even offering it as a potential solution would have the biggest chance of me probably using it.[d]

This suggests the possibility of using online peer networks as a gateway to facilitate young people's access to offline support where they need this.

It can, however, be misleading to assume that because some young people feel comfortable in online contexts, this is true for all young people. Ito cautions against an approach which assumes that all young people are immersed in digital communication, and certainly in our research we heard from a relatively small number of young people who were not comfortable with using this medium of communication to talk about intimate or sensitive issues.[103] Some of the differences we see in this may be due to cultural beliefs. One young Pacific Island woman, for example, captured how she felt less comfortable about putting herself and her own needs forward in this way:

> You go online and you're like 'oh, here's a way to... for yourself' cause everyone's different you know, everyone is going to get better differently or feel safe differently and I think that... especially for PI's [Pacific Islanders], it's ... they're real humble. They don't want to tell people they're upset. They don't want to make themselves a priority to someone else so ... you don't find any help on social media or anywhere for us.[d]

Despite these exceptions, it does appear that young people are trying to find and provide support in their own social media networks. Their practices, however, suggest that they may have priorities that are not always sufficiently acknowledged in the design of professional online resources. It is clear that young people approach online support, even in their own networks, with the same caution we see in their other relationships. They know there are risks in making themselves vulnerable online. It is not enough for them to have anonymity and accurate information. Young people are looking for trust, relational connection, and affirmation in their support seeking. They are also looking for respect for their agency and sensitivity to their individual needs. There is much that professionals can learn from young people's informal online peer support practices in their design of professional interventions in this new terrain.

What do young people want?

Young people want digital support that recognises their fundamental needs for trust and connection. This support also needs to accommodate young people's agency and individuality, recognising that they are active participants in finding and creating the resources they want online.

Those working with young people can help by

- Empowering them to manage their emotional safety online.
- Facilitating young people's ability to support one another online.
- Recognising the advantages of online support including anonymity, ease of access, and privacy.
- Prioritising online resources that offer a relational connection.
- Supporting them to find or develop those online resources that best meet their needs.

9 A Youth Informed Approach to mental health

Throughout this book, I have tried to capture the world that young people live in today and how this influences their priorities for mental health support. But lurking beneath the clear voices of the young people we interviewed in our research is the spectre of a clunky, outdated, and unresponsive mental health system which, in many cases, has remained unchanged for decades. It is, perhaps, little wonder that young people are reluctant to use these mental health resources. For too long we have made only minor adjustments to cater for the needs of our younger clients, with small changes that accommodate what we think of as their 'developmental needs.'; The problem is that conceptualisations of young people, drawing as they do from outdated ideas of what youth looks like, do not capture the significant changes in society, families, and technology that have helped to shape the lives of young people differently in this generation. It is time to develop a better approach to youth mental health that recognises the strengths of young people as well as the challenges they face. We need a way of engaging with youth that can fit with the needs of this digital-savvy generation who know what they want from mental health services and recognise when they are not getting it.

It is not necessary to have a blueprint or a manual for 'how to do therapy' with young people. There are indeed so many competing approaches, most with strong evidence to support their effectiveness, that it would be impossible to single out one 'right' way of working therapeutically with young people experiencing distress.[154] Nonetheless it is helpful to establish core principles that can guide practitioners, service managers, and policymakers towards an overarching approach which can better meet the needs of young people today. This can be thought of in much the same way as the, well-known, *trauma-informed care* model which sets out to make services safe for people who have experienced trauma by looking at everything from the reception, the setting, and the tone of the engagement to the intervention approach itself.[155] Borrowing from this terminology, I have called this a *Youth Informed Approach* (YIA). A Youth Informed Approach has a number of key principles which are outlined below.

DOI: 10.4324/9780429322457-9

Principle one: Normalise distress and help-seeking

With stigma being one of the most profound barriers to young people accessing mental health support it is important to de-pathologise mental health problems. Attempts to do this by likening mental health problems to physical health problems have not been successful and in some cases might increase stigma. Talking about mental health problems in supposedly neutral diagnostic terms can also backfire as these labels pose significant challenges to young people's developing identity during a period in which this is fundamental.

To de-pathologise mental health distress, it is important to use diagnostic labels sparingly and avoid them where possible, especially with the more common and milder mental health problems that usually fall under the label of 'depression' or 'anxiety.' While young people may be drawn to mental health labels themselves, the benefit of using this to reassure them that their distress is valid and that they are deserving of help needs to be weighed against the longer-term impacts on their sense of self and future well-being. It is possible to convey to young people that their problems are 'real' and 'valid' without using diagnostic labels and instead by recognising that distress is an understandable response to the challenges they face. This approach fits well with the broader shifts away from diagnostic approaches to assessment and treatment in the field of psychology.

In much the same way, the act of seeking help needs to be normalised and de-medicalised. Talking about distress and asking for help should be reclaimed as a legitimate way for young people to find support during difficult times without their having to prove they have some sort of 'illness' which justifies this.

Principle two: *Tailor support to identity*

For young people, the making of identity is a central task and challenges to this are often at the heart of their distress. The experience of having mental health difficulties and of seeking help can also have a profound effect on young people's developing sense of who they are. For this reason, it is important to recognise the particular significance of identity in all our efforts to support young people struggling with distress.

The way we offer and provide support to different groups of young people needs to be matched to those aspects of their identity which are important to them. These aspects of identity may include their culture or ethnicity, their religion, their sexuality, or gender. It is tempting to slip into making generalisations about what sorts of approaches are appropriate for these different collective identities, but as young people's sense of themselves tends to be more fluid and idiosyncratic in this generation it is difficult to know exactly which aspects of identity matter to a young person without asking them. The advice service users give to clinicians is relevant here: 'Ask who are you?' before asking: 'What is wrong with you?' Finding out who a young person is in counselling and helping them to do the same, is likely to be as important as addressing their symptoms.

It is also vital to take into account, the damaging effects of mental health stigma on young people's developing identity. This can be counteracted by facilitating more validating and compassionate views of people experiencing mental health difficulties, both with individual clients and within society more broadly.

Principle three: *Respect choice*

It is crucial to respect young people's agency. This is more than just an internal 'developmental' need but rather reflects the position that young people often occupy in society; on the one hand being asked to take on more responsibility and on the other hand being denied access to real power. The frustrations that young people feel about their lack of power in society are an understandable response to this contradictory set of expectations.

For young people to be willing to engage with the support they need to be treated as equals and with respect. Young people should be allowed to make their own choices about when and where to seek help, in all but the most extreme cases where there are imminent risks to their safety. The costs of forcing young people to see a professional for 'their own good' far outweigh any benefit these kinds of interventions might be thought to have.

Within the counselling setting itself, young people should also be given choices about the kind of help they want. In addition, mental health professionals need to remain conscious of their own power in these situations. Mental health professionals may need to work actively to empower young clients to help them to express their opinions, recognising that there may be constraints on this that are not always visible to those who hold the power.

Principle four: *Listen more than talk*

There is a temptation for adults to give advice to youth from a position that assumes they have 'been through it' and have more knowledge about what would be best. But given the profound changes that have taken place over the past decades, it is important to realise that being older is no guarantee of being right. Young people need to be able to talk openly about the things that matter to them, including sensitive issues like suicide. Adults need to be willing to adopt a respectful listening attitude to young people and open their eyes to understand their world, what they value, and the challenges they face.

This listening stance translates well into the counselling environment, where young people will benefit from the opportunity to articulate and reflect on their experiences, drawing their own conclusions about the sort of life they want to lead. While professionals often feel pressure to have the answer, especially when faced with a young person in distress, it is almost always more helpful to allow young people to explore potential solutions for themselves.

While the emphasis in recent models of therapy has been on the need to 'regulate emotions' or to challenge unhelpful thinking, the opportunity for young people to simply express themselves in a safe space provides an important antidote to the constraints on what they feel able to express in their outside lives.

Principle five: *Build trusting relationships*

It is clear that young people in this generation continue to value relationships as much, if not more so, than previous generations. Given young people's heightened awareness of the potential for being manipulated through false information and inauthentic relationships, trust has taken on particular importance.

Trust is a necessary prerequisite for young people being able to talk about their distress or to receive help. This applies in professional counselling relationships as much as it does in the informal networks that young people often use for support. The development of trusting relationships takes time and young people cannot be expected to simply confide their distress to a professional. They are much more likely to talk to a friend or an adult with whom they have an existing relationship of trust.

Recognising the importance of trust for young people also has implications for the way in which we provide formal counselling support. The standard model, in which we expect a young person to confide their distress to a stranger within the first hour of meeting, needs to be revised. Instead, we need to look at how young people can be introduced to formal support in more gradual ways that allow them to build relationships before they are asked to talk about their problems. In the same vein, we need to prioritise providing young people with ongoing relationships with a mental health professional and stop the practice of moving them from one clinician or service to another.

Principle six: *Utilise informal social networks*

Regardless of the way that professional services are set up, most young people will still tend to rely on their peers for support. These informal peer networks operate online as well as in real life. It is important not to romanticise peer relationships, and some young people's difficulties happen specifically in these friendship groups. Nonetheless, for many young people, these are the mainstay of their well-being. These peer support networks need to be recognised as a valuable part of the day-to-day support surrounding young people. Professionals can help by encouraging young people to develop these supportive peer networks in healthy ways and recognising them as an important part of their lives. There are also opportunities to mobilise these networks to facilitate young people's access to counselling or to help them navigate the process of receiving help or recovery.

Young people's relationships with their families can be complicated at this point in their lives. While family support matters to young people, these relationships might also challenge their need for agency and privacy. As with friendship groups, families can also be a significant source of young people's difficulties. It is important when considering the role of families for young people to be guided in individual situations by the personal or cultural appropriateness of actively including these networks in any intervention. It would be best, where possible, to provide young people with the primary choice in relation to this and it may not be appropriate to routinely include all family members in an initial therapy session with a young client. Where young people are reluctant to have their families involved, it may be more fruitful to gradually explore the potential for making a space for family involvement with the agreement of, and at a pace suitable for, the young client. In more collectivist cultures, such as Māori and Pacific Islanders, the advantages of this approach will need to be weighed against the potential to undermine the cultural value given to family involvement.

Counsellors or other professionals will have limitations on their availability, whereas these informal support networks are available 24 hours a day and can provide a sense of belonging which bolsters young people's ongoing capacity to deal with challenges.

Principle seven: *Improve accessibility*

Mental health support should consider young people's preference to be able to access support when and where they need it. Many of the formal mental health services are difficult for young people to access and do not fit well around their lives.

Young people need physical services that they can access easily without having to travel far away or pay a lot of money. These services need to be located in places that young people already congregate. Counselling services in schools and universities are valuable to young people, but as these options are not available or acceptable to all young people there need to be youth counselling services in local communities. While typically these services have been sited alongside or together with other health services for young people, it may be more helpful to align them to community youth centres which have a broader purpose and which will contribute to normalising help-seeking.

It is vitally important that young people can access these services easily on their own and are not reliant on adults around them to mediate this on their behalf. They need to be able to make appointments independently and should be supported and encouraged to do this when they need to. Young people should also not have to wait for long periods for appointments and ideally there need to be some walk-in appointments available for them in their moment of need.

Where possible, it would be valuable to separate youth services out from services which are designed for young children, challenging the common tendency to combine these into a 'child and adolescent' service. The premises from which the services operate need to be made youth-friendly, including spaces designed to match youth priorities for informality. Young people need to feel welcomed into these spaces from their first encounter with the waiting space, their dealings with the receptionist, and the consulting room itself.

Principle eight: *Use technology*

While digital technology is not a panacea for all youth mental health needs, it does have an important part to play in adding to the support options available to young people. However, it is important that these interventions and resources are developed with young people's own priorities and digital practices in mind.

Building on young people's familiarity and comfort with digital communication, it is valuable to utilise this to help them make sense of their difficulties, access psycho-educational resources, and receive support. Ideally, these interventions should create some space for personal contact with a 'real' person who can provide a sense of relational connection. Online intervention developers should also recognise the importance of trust for young people in engaging with these online resources. Well-known youth providers might offer some reassurance of safety, and it can be useful to also draw on personal friend networks and social media influencers to facilitate young people's access to appropriate online support.

While it is important to provide these resources, it is also vital to recognise that young people's preferences for online mental health support might be less controllable and predictable than professionals tend to think. Young people are more likely to pick and choose what they need from formal and informal resources and use these in idiosyncratic and creative ways to meet their own unique needs. It may be most helpful for professionals to recognise this potential and support young people to safely negotiate the vast array of resources available online and to find those that work best for them.

While the internet does contain dangers for young people, it is important not to demonise this medium but to rather work with young people to explore how they can protect themselves against the emotional risks entailed in being online and make the most of the potential for meaningful support and engagement.

Principle nine: *Allow inclusive decision making*

Given young people's expertise in their own lives and their awareness of the opportunities and challenges in this digital age, it is important to include them as participants in addressing their own mental health needs. We need to listen to young people's views about important issues like youth suicide, social media, and climate change. We need to take seriously the way that they understand youth mental health and use this to supplement our own understandings as adults and professionals. We also need to listen to their ideas about what kinds of support work well for them, which do not, and how we can improve mental health services more generally.

Beyond simply hearing what young people say, we need to include them in decision-making bodies and processes that will influence the development of services and the design of interventions.

Promising directions in youth mental health

While many mental health services continue to remain stuck in the past, there are several innovative youth mental health models being developed around the world. Some of these models have been translated into youth-friendly services including headspace in Australia, Jigsaw in Ireland, Maisons des Adolescents in France, Foundry in Canada and what are called Youth One Stop Shops in New Zealand.[2] These developments are part of a growing recognition of the need to replace the outdated services available for young people with resources that offer appropriate early intervention for this hard to reach population.

Sarah Hetrick together with colleagues from other countries summarised the results of service evaluations that had been conducted by these youth-friendly services to try and establish those aspects that young people particularly valued.[156] The features that young people appreciated in these services fit well with many of the principles outlined in the YIA approach. They include that services were easily accessible and that they were welcoming and informal. The evaluations also highlighted the value of having relationships with those who worked at the service and also having other young people as part of the staff. In addition, young clients appreciated that appointments were made in a timely manner, that these were provided at low cost, and that interventions were appropriate and safe. The evaluations also noted the importance of maintaining young clients' needs for privacy and confidentiality. The authors of this article also underlined the significance of stigma noting, for example, that young people preferred not having clinical signage that made the services too 'medical.' The only area of significant difference with the YIA approach was in the recommendation for the integration of physical and mental health, which might reflect the overarching primary health care model which provided the framework for many of the services evaluated.

While these youth-friendly services represent a very hopeful direction for addressing young people's mental health needs, there are still further challenges ahead. Many of the services that exist were developed as prototypes and have not been systematically rolled out across the countries in which they have been developed. Some of these also rely on somewhat erratic funding arrangements. Even headspace, which has an extensive network of centres across Australia, is dependent on the whims of the current government to see whether they can expand to meet the needs of young people.[157] In New Zealand, the 11 centres identified as Youth One Stop Shops have been very responsive to their local communities but lack reliable funding and consistency of model.[158]

There are also some exciting new youth-friendly online services and resources being developed alongside these face-to-face initiatives. Many counselling services provided to young people through youth services or university clinics now offer an online option as an addition to their face-to-face services. These can offer access to group or individual counsellors or even provide careful mental health assessments. These online resources have the potential to provide support to young people living in remote areas or with other constraints on their ability to access services, provided they have access to the appropriate technology.[159] Online support can also be offered as a way of bridging support in the time that young people might have to wait to be seen face-to-face. Counsellors are also starting to use a variety of apps as an adjunct to face-to-face counselling, providing continuity of connection between sessions and facilitating discussions with clients about their experiences within the session.[160]

More innovative online interventions have tried to reach out proactively to the online spaces in which young people are already interacting. *Live for Tomorrow* is a unique service that relies on volunteer counsellors (young people themselves) to respond by message to posts that suggest suicidality on Instagram.[161] These kinds of interventions have the potential to overcome the barriers that prevent young people from seeking professional help online as well as offline.

The value of these services is dependent on increased recognition and appropriate funding in their host countries and internationally. In addition, the existing outline of an appropriate service model for addressing youth mental health still requires further elaboration. The details of how these innovative models can work for young people rely on understanding better what young people themselves want. It is also important to continue to develop these initiatives in a way that matches the ongoing changes in young people's worlds.

While there is increasing recognition of the need to gather young people's evaluations of services and to use these to inform their development, the approach to evaluation research is sometimes limited.[156] Firstly, evaluations often call on young people to comment on a service which is already in operation. This limits the involvement they can have in the development of services and also tends to elicit reactions to what *is* rather than exploring the full range of what might be possible. Secondly, evaluations tend to rely on eliciting the views of only the young people who have actually used a service and in this way excludes the voices of those who may not have felt comfortable to do so. Sometimes, these evaluations might also unwittingly reflect the need to impress funders with measurable outcomes, support for feasibility or low cost, rather than having the primary objective of capturing young people's experiences and opinions. Furthermore, these kinds of evaluations tend to focus on features of the service itself rather than exploring young people's priorities in the broader context of their lives. This can render important aspects of young people's lives and mental health invisible to service providers and policy makers. Furthermore, many service user evaluation studies rely on questionnaires with fixed option responses and might not always allow young people the opportunity to share their knowledge or demonstrate their ability to think outside the box. Finally, the power dynamics that operate between young people and researchers might also limit their ability to have their voices heard.[162] Jessica Stubbing and I recently tried out a new workshop method for exploring young people's hopes and dreams for a mental health service. This offered those who took part in the workshops an opportunity to discuss and debate with their peers and demonstrated their ability to generate creative ideas for engaging young people with mental health support.[o]

There is also a growing awareness of the importance of including young people in the design of interventions with some excellent models being used to do this with online mental health resources. The #Chatsafe project led by Jo Robinson and her team at Orygen, which provides young people with guidelines on how to talk safely about suicide, for example, was developed with the help of young people.[163] It is important here, as with evaluation studies, that we not only include young people as commentators on existing designs and services but also learn more about their online preferences and practices and use these as a starting point for co-designing support.

Encouragingly, young people are increasingly being called on to play a role in organisations which support youth mental health.[18] Peer support networks are being more widely recognised as a useful resource, both on[164] and offline.[165] There is also growing recognition of the need for youth representation in the decision making of mental health services. On an international level, the need for youth-friendly services with youth involvement has been recognised in the 2012 establishment of the International Association of Youth Mental Health, a connecting body formed under the leadership of Patrick McGorry, the Director of Orygen Youth Health and the Orygen Youth Health Research Centre in Australia.

Despite these reassuring initiatives, there is a danger that the imbalance of power between young people and adult professionals play out in these forums the way it might in the consulting room. It is important to ensure that young people are represented in sufficient numbers to provide them with the confidence to voice their opinions and that adult professionals are aware of, and challenge, the way that they might hold power, in ways that they may not always fully realise.

Training mental health professionals differently

While lack of recognition of young people's voices, and lack of funding for initiatives to support them, lie at the root of the slowness in the pace of change, it is perhaps surprising that one of the most significant challenges to transformation in youth mental health services come from mental health professionals themselves. Most mental health workers who are involved with young people are passionate about their work and see the importance of engaging with young people, but it can be difficult for them to abandon the conventions that underlie their approach to working with young people and give up the professional power associated with their established roles. Professional training tends also to be mired in these same systems and while fashions in models change, the basic ways of working have often been left unchallenged.

Many clinicians have also been caught up in contemporary concerns to provide evidence-based interventions that focus on symptom change. While this has value for their work and their clients, the concern to identify efficacious interventions and use these reliably has sometimes been at the expense of some of the foundations of counselling. New clinicians need to be trained to recognise the importance of seeing and adapting to the client in front of them rather than focusing on pre-determined strategies and techniques. The certainty of manualised approaches, or a pre-determined session plan, is appealing to inexperienced clinicians, but they need to be taught to get to know their client, to find out what works for them and what they want to get out of any support relationship.

Young professionals also need reminding of the fundamental value of the relationship in counselling and be taught to recognise the importance of slowly developing a trusting connection before any meaningful work can be done. In addition, mental health professionals need to extend their gaze beyond the consulting room and to develop their understanding of constraints of the social context in which young people struggle to find power. They also need to remain aware of their own position, and the power this holds.

We need to train professionals who can better understand the diversity of young clients we engage with. One of the things we need to do is to train more clinicians from minority groups so that young people can work with someone of their own culture, gender, or sexuality if they prefer this. We would also do well to draw from the extensive literature on culture-sensitive approaches to counselling to be able to work across all sorts of cultural differences, including those differences that exist between the cultures of adult professionals and youth.[166] In addition, it would be valuable to explore ways of providing training to young people who do not fit the criteria for access to professional training but can nonetheless provide important youth-friendly support to other young people.

Engagement with digital technology has posed a particular challenge to mental health professionals whose approach to these often varies somewhere between ambivalent and reluctant. I have been in many settings where professionals have raised concerns about shifts towards online interventions. Their objections usually relate to ethical issues and the difficulties of ensuring the safety of young clients online.[167] This is a legitimate concern, but it is difficult to justify the decision to close their professional eyes to the many young people who are willing to talk about suicide online in the interest of ensuring that established safety protocols can be followed. We need to develop new guidelines for how to manage our professional responsibilities for risk in online environments that recognise that we are working in a context where there is less ability to control the situation than we are used to.

Professionals' other major objection to online support arises from their fear of losing a relational connection with their clients. These objections can, however, be addressed by helping professionals to understand young people's preference for relationality in their online interactions and supporting them to build meaningful relationships with their clients in these spaces.

Professionals also raise concerns about the potential for online work to challenge established boundaries between clinicians and their clients and perhaps also challenge their own preferences for working nine to five. Ultimately, some of the professional anxiety about using or supporting online resources might have more to do with professionals' anxieties about being forced to work in an area in which they are less confident and skilled. It would be important to offer training in this area to new and established practitioners if we want to have their help in engaging young people via this medium.

Allowing space to change

The argument at the heart of this book is that we need to shift our ways of working to match the changes that have shaped the experiences of young people today. Following this line of thinking, it must be recognised that in order to reach young people in distress, we will need to respond to evolving and new contexts. Just as we feel we have understood youth today, we may need to update ourselves to changes in the context and priorities of young people.

As I complete this book, we are living through the dramatic transformations that COVID-19 has wrought on much of what we considered to be 'normal' society. We have experienced the way the world as we know it can be turned upside down in a very short amount of time. With countries facing the threat or actuality of large-scale illness, the breakdown of health services and rolling periods of lockdown, the toll on youth mental health has already been identified as a significant concern. It is beyond the scope of this book to write about the effects this has had on young people's well-being or the way it might impact on their future, but it has certainly underlined the potential for those aspects of the environment that young people find difficult, to become even worse, exacerbating young people's feelings of isolation, their concern for their future, and handing them a world that seems fraught with uncertainty and dissent.

The pandemic has, however, had one rather unexpected helpful outcome and that is the normalisation of distress and the reminder that this is often a legitimate response to circumstances rather than a weakness in an individual. This allows young people to be given the more helpful message that 'it is okay to not be okay.' This may provide an opportunity to challenge the stigma surrounding mental health and to encourage greater acceptance of the challenges facing young people today.

The importance of technology in helping people communicate has also never been so well recognised as it has during this period. Older people are finally catching up to young people in their recognition of the value of social media as a way of connecting with others as Zoom has begun to mediate everyone's work and social interactions. Ironically, as this occurs, both young and old seem more aware than ever of the limitations of online communication as the option of face-to-face contact is temporarily removed from them. Besides the immediate impacts of the pandemic, young people will continue to live through the economic and social damage it will leave in its wake. The dramatic changes we have seen in this short period also give us a taste of the potential for other large-scale changes that might be brought about the further pandemics, political upheaval, or climate change.

All these contextual changes bring out transformations in youth cultures, different ways of understanding mental health and different priorities and concerns young people have about engaging with support. We cannot predict these future changes but need to hold on to the importance of adopting an approach to youth mental health which recognises and responds to what young people want.

Data Sources

a. "A qualitative exploration of adolescents' views of seeking help when experiencing stress." Ethics approval from the University of Auckland Human Participants Ethics Committee, 2014. Researchers: Emma Edwards and Kerry Gibson (supervisor). Data previously published in:
Edwards, Emma. 2016. ""We're all in the same boat": Views and experiences of stress, coping and help-seeking among New Zealand youth". DClinPsy thesis, University of Auckland.

b. "Young people's talk about suicide: Identifying risk and resilience." Ethics approval from the University of Auckland Human Participants Ethics Com mittee, 2015. Researchers: Kerry Gibson, Fred Seymour, Jan Wilson, and Margaret Wetherell. Funder: Oakley Mental Health Foundation. Data previously published in:
Gibson, Kerry, Jan Wilson, Jade Le Grice, and Fred Seymour. 2019 "Resisting the silence: The impact of digital communication on young people's talk about suicide." *Youth & Society* 51(8):1011–1030.
Stubbing, Jessica, and Kerry Gibson. 2019. "Young people's explanations for youth suicide in New Zealand: A thematic analysis." *Journal of Youth Studies* 22 (4): 520–532. Stubbing, Jessica. 2017. "Young people's perspectives on the reasons for youth suicide in New Zealand". Psychology Honours diss., University of Auckland.

c. "A qualitative exploration of how Chinese migrant youths cope with stress in New Zealand." Ethics approval from University of Auckland Human Participants Ethics Committee, 2013. Researchers: Yan Yan Lei and Kerry Gibson (supervisor). Data previously published in:
Lei, Yan Yan. 2016. "A qualitative exploration of stress, coping, support-seeking, and help-seeking among Chinese migrant youth in New Zealand." DClinPsy thesis, University of Auckland.

d. "Improving youth mental health: Finding support safely on the internet." Ethics approval from University of Auckland Human Participants Ethics Committee, 2019. Researchers: Kerry Gibson and Susanna Trnka. Funders: Internet
New Zealand. Data previously published in:
Adeane, Emily. 2020. "Online messages, offline help: Using the internet to connect young people to psychological Support." Psychology Honours diss., University of Auckland.

e. "An analysis of young people's posts to an internet suicide prevention forum." No ethics approval required. Researchers: Aamina Ali and Kerry Gibson (supervisor). Data previously published in:
Ali, Aamina. 2015. "Reasons young people provide for feeling suicidal." Psychology Honours diss., University of Auckland. Ali, Aamina, and Kerry Gibson. 2019. "Young people's reasons for feeling suicidal: An analysis of posts to a social media suicide prevention forum." *Crisis: The Journal of Crisis Intervention and Suicide Prevention* 40:400–406.

f. "Stressors and coping mechanisms of Kiwi Muslim youth." Ethics approval from University of Auckland Human Participants Ethics Committee, 2013. Researchers: Aamina Ali and Kerry Gibson (supervisor). Data previously published in:
Ali, Aamina. 2019. "Psychological stress and coping in adolescent Muslim New Zealanders: A key informant perspective." DClinPsy thesis, University of Auckland.

g. "Peer support online: An exploration of how young people give and receive support for psychological distress: Survey". Ethics approval from University of Auckland Human Participants Ethics Committee, 2017. Researchers Kerry Gibson and Susanna Trnka. Funders: University of Auckland, Faculty of Science Research Development Fund. Data previously published in:
Nasier, Bilal. 2019. ""PM me": Young peoples' perceptions of supportive versus unsympathetic responses to distress online." Psychology Honours diss., University of Auckland.

h. "Young women talk about their experiences of taking antidepressants". Ethics approval from University of Auckland Human Participants Ethics Committee, 2012. Researchers Celine Wills and Kerry Gibson (supervisor). Data previously published in:
Wills, Celine. 2015. ""A hard pill to swallow": Young women's experiences of taking antidepressants. DClinPsy thesis, University of Auckland.
Wills, Celine, Kerry Gibson, Claire Cartwright, and John Read. 2019. "Young women's selfhood on antidepressants: "Not fully myself"." *Qualitative Health Research* 30 (2):268–278.

i. "Peer support online: An exploration of how young people give and receive support for psychological distress: Instant messaging interviews". Ethics approval from University of Auckland Human Participants Ethics Committee, 2017. Researchers Kerry Gibson and Susanna Trnka. Funders: University of Auckland, Faculty of Science Research Development Fund. Data previously published in:
Gibson, Kerry, and Susanna Trnka. 2020. "Young people's priorities for support on social media: "It takes trust to talk about these issues"." *Computers in Human Behavior* 102: 238–247.

j. "Young people talk about their experiences of telephone and text counselling." Ethics approval from University of Auckland Human Participants Ethics Committee, 2012. Researchers: Kerry Gibson and Claire Cartwright. Funders: University of Auckland, Faculty of Science Research Development Fund. Data previously published in:
Campbell, Julia. 2014. "I think I am what I am because of that phone call: Young people talk about their experience of telephone counselling." Psychology Honours diss., University of Auckland. Gibson, Kerry, and Claire Cartwright. 2014. "Young people's experiences of mobile phone text counselling: Balancing connection and control." *Children and Youth Services Review* 43: 96–104.
Gibson, Kerry, Claire Cartwright, Kelly Kerrisk, Julia Campbell, and Fred

Seymour. 2016. "What young people want: A qualitative study of adolescents' priorities for engagement across psychological services." *Journal of Child and Family Studies* 25 (4): 1057–1065.

k. "Looking back, making sense: Narratives of youth mental health problems and recovery." Ethics approval from University of Auckland Human Participants Ethics Committee, 2015. Researchers Rebecca Herald and Kerry Gibson (supervisor). Data previously published in:
Herald, Rebecca. 2019. ""How I got here": Personal narratives of youth mental health difficulties and recovery." DClinPsy thesis, University of Auckland.

l. "Young people talk about their experiences of psychological counselling." Ethics Approval from the Health and Disability Ethics Committee, 2013. Researchers Kelly Kerrisk and Kerry Gibson (supervisor). Data previously published in:
Kerrisk, Kelly. 2014. "Narrative, identity, and meaning making: Young people's experiences of psychotherapy." DClinPsy thesis, University of Auckland.
Gibson, Kerry, Claire Cartwright, Kelly Kerrisk, Julia Campbell, and Fred Seymour. 2016. "What young people want: A qualitative study of adolescents' priorities for engagement across psychological services." *Journal of Child and Family Studies* 25 (4): 1057–1065.

m. "Young people talk about their experiences of psychological assessment." Ethics Approval from the Health and Disability Ethics Committee, 2013. Researchers: Ting-ya Wang and Kerry Gibson (supervisor). Data previously published in:
Wang, T. (2014). "Young people's experiences of assessment in a mental health setting." DClinPsy thesis, University of Auckland.

n. "Adolescents' accounts of their journey through psychological counselling." Ethics Approval from the Health and Disability Ethics Committee, 2012. Researcher: Kerry Gibson. Funders: University of Auckland, Faculty of Science Research Development Fund. Data previously published in:
Gibson, Kerry, and Claire Cartwright, C. 2013. "Agency in young clients' narratives of counseling: "It's whatever you want to make of it"." *Journal of Counseling Psychology* 60 (3):340–352.
Gibson, Kerry, Claire Cartwright, Kelly Kerrisk, Julia Campbell, and Fred Seymour. 2016. "What young people want: A qualitative study of adolescents' priorities for engagement across psychological services." *Journal of Child and Family Studies* 25 (4):1057–1065.
Knight, Karis, Kerry Gibson, and Claire Cartwright. 2018. ""It's like a refuge": Young people's relationships with school counsellors." *Counselling and Psychotherapy Research* 18 (4): 345–411.
Knight, Karis, 2017. "Young people and the therapeutic relationship." Psychology Honours diss., University of Auckland.

o. "What do young people want? Designing mental health services in New Zealand." Ethics approval from University of Auckland Human Participants Ethics Committee, 2018. Researchers Jessica Stubbing and Kerry Gibson (supervisor). Data previously published in:
Stubbing, Jessica. 2021. ""Nobody has ever asked me that": Reimagining mental health care through collaborative research with young people from New Zealand." DClinPsy thesis, University of Auckland.

p. "An analysis of young people's suicide conversations on a text counselling service." Ethics approval from University of Auckland Human Participants

Ethics Committee, 2016. Researchers: Jeanne Van Wyk and Kerry Gibson (supervisor). Data previously published in:
Van Wyk, Jeanne. 2021. ""I'm scared of what i might do to myself": Young people's communication about suicide on a text message counselling service." DClinPsy thesis, University of Auckland.

q. "Ka hao te rangatahi: Fishing with a new net? Rethinking responsibility for youth mental health in the digital age". Ethics approval from the University of Auckland Human Participants Ethics Committee, 2020. Researchers: Susanna Trnka, Kerry Gibson, Monique Jonas Pikihuia Pomare, and Jemaima Tiatia-Seath. Funders: Marsden Fund – Royal Society of New Zealand.

References

1 Patel, Vikram, Alan J Flisher, Sarah Hetrick, and Patrick McGorry. 2007. "Mental health of young people: A global public-health challenge." *The Lancet* 369 (9569):1302–1313.

2 McGorry, Patrick, Tony Bates, and Max Birchwood. 2013. "Designing youth mental health services for the 21st century: Examples from Australia, Ireland and the UK." *The British Journal of Psychiatry* 202 (s54):s30–s35.

3 Woodman, Dan, and Johanna Wyn. 2014. *Youth and generation: Rethinking change and inequality in the lives of young people.* London: Sage.

4 Wyn, Johanna, and Anita Harris. 2004. "Youth research in Australia and New Zealand." *Young* 12(3):271–289.

5 Landstedt, Evelina, Julia Coffey, Johanna Wyn, Hernán Cuervo, and Dan Woodman. 2017. "The complex relationship between mental health and social conditions in the lives of young Australians mixing work and study." *Young* 25(4):339–358.

6 Cuervo, Hernán, and Johanna Wyn. 2011. *Rethinking youth transitions in Australia: A historical and multidimensional approach.* Research Report 33. Melbourne: Youth Research Centre, University of Melbourne.

7 Beck, Ulrich, and Elisabeth Beck-Gernsheim. 2001. *Individualization: Institutionalized individualism and its social and political consequences.* London, United Kingdom: Sage Publications.

8 Furlong, Andy, and Fred Cartmel. 2007. *Young people and social change: New perspectives.* Maidenhead: Open University Press.

9 White, Rob. 2011. "Climate change, uncertain futures and the sociology of youth." *Youth Studies Australia* 30(3):13.

10 Arnett, Jeffrey Jensen. 2007. "Emerging adulthood: What is it, and what is it good for?" *Child Development Perspectives* 1 (2):68–73.

11 United Nations. 2013. "Definition of youth." *United Nations.* Accessed 25 February 2021. Retrieved from https://www.un.org/esa/socdev/documents/youth/fact-sheets/youth-definition.pdf.

12 Johnson, Sara B, Robert W Blum, and Jay N Giedd. 2009. "Adolescent maturity and the brain: The promise and pitfalls of neuroscience research in adolescent health policy." *Journal of Adolescent Health* 45 (3):216–221.

13 Wellplace.nz. "Who's drinking and how much." *Wellplace.nz.* Accessed 25 February 2021. Retrieved from https://wellplace.nz/facts-and-information/alcohol/drinking-in-new-zealand/.

14 Helman, Cecil. 2000. *Culture, health and illness.* 4th ed. London: Arnold.

15 Hall, G Stanley. 1904. *Adolescence: Its psychology and its relations to physiology, anthropology, sociology, sex, crime, religion, and education.* New York: D. Appleton and Company.

16 Marsh, Ian. 2015. "Critiquing contemporary suicidology." In *Critical suicidology: Transforming suicide research and prevention for the 21st century*, edited by Jennifer White, Ian Marsh, Michael J Kral and Jonathan Morris. Toronto, Ontario, Canada: UBC Press.

17 Longdon, Eleanor, and John Read. 2017. "'People with problems, not patients with illnesses': Using psychosocial frameworks to reduce the stigma of psychosis." *Israel Journal of Psychiatry and Related Sciences* 54(1):24–30.

18 Coughlan, Helen, Mary Cannon, David Shiers, Paddy Power, Claire Barry, Tony Bates, Max Birchwood, Sarah Buckley, Derek Chambers, and Simon Davidson.

2013. "Towards a new paradigm of care: The International Declaration on Youth Mental Health." *Early Intervention in Psychiatry* 2 (7):103–108.

19 Furlong, Andy, Dan Woodman, and Johanna Wyn. 2011. "Changing times, changing perspectives: Reconciling 'transition' and 'cultural' perspectives on youth and young adulthood." *Journal of Sociology* 47 (4):355–370.

20 Hodkinson, Paul. 2016. "Youth cultures and the rest of life: Subcultures, post-subcultures and beyond." *Journal of Youth Studies* 19 (5):629–645.

21 Markovits, Daniel. 2019. *The meritocracy trap*. New York: Penguin UK.

22 UNICEF. 2017. *Building the future: Children and the sustainable development goals in rich countries.* Innocenti Report Card 14. Florence: UNICEF Office of Research, Innocenti.

23 O'Neill, Anne-Marie. 2016. "Assessment-based curriculum: Globalising and enterprising culture, human capital and teacher–technicians in Aotearoa New Zealand." *Journal of Education Policy* 31 (5):598–621.

24 Rodway, Cathryn, Su-Gwan Tham, Saied Ibrahim, Pauline Turnbull, Kirsten Windfuhr, Jenny Shaw, Nav Kapur, and Louis Appleby. 2016. "Suicide in children and young people in England: A consecutive case series." *The Lancet Psychiatry* 3 (8):751–759.

25 Cuervo, Hernan, and Johanna Wyn. 2016. "An unspoken crisis: The 'scarring effects' of the complex nexus between education and work on two generations of young Australians." *International Journal of Lifelong Education* 35 (2):122–135.

26 Cuervo, Hernán, and Johanna Wyn. 2014. "Reflections on the use of spatial and relational metaphors in youth studies." *Journal of Youth Studies* 17 (7):901–915.

27 Cotterell, John. 2007. *Social networks in youth and adolescence.* East Sussex: Routledge.

28 Collins, W Andrew. 2003. "More than myth: The developmental significance of romantic relationships during adolescence." *Journal of Research on Adolescence* 13 (1):1–24.

29 Cuervo, Hernán, and Jun Fu. 2020. "Rethinking family relationships." In *Youth and the new adulthood: Generations of change*, edited byJohanna Wyn, Helen Cahill, Dan Woodman, Hernán Cuervo, Carmen Leccardi and Jenny Chesters, 99–114. Singapore: Springer Singapore.

30 Haidt, Jonathan, and Greg Lukianoff. 2018. *The coddling of the American mind: How good intentions and bad ideas are setting up a generation for failure.* New York: Penguin UK.

31 Noller, Patricia, and Sharon Atkin. 2014. *Family life in adolescence.* Warsaw, Poland, Berlin, Germany: De Gruyter Open.

32 Cook, Julia, and Katherine Romei. 2020. "Belonging, place and entrepreneurial selfhood." In *Youth and the new adulthood: Generations of change*, edited by Johanna Wyn, Helen Cahill, Dan Woodman, Hernán Cuervo, Carmen Leccardi and Jenny Chesters, 83–97. Singapore: Springer Singapore.

33 Crosnoe, Robert. 2011. *Fitting in, standing out: Navigating the social challenges of high school to get an education.* New York: Cambridge University Press.

34 Johnson, Corey W, Anneliese A Singh, and Maru Gonzalez. 2014. ""It's complicated": Collective memories of transgender, queer, and questioning youth in high school." *Journal of Homosexuality* 61 (3):419–434.

35 Porcelli, Paola, Michael Ungar, Linda Liebenberg, and Nathalie Trépanier. 2014. "(Micro) mobility, disability and resilience: Exploring well-being among youth with physical disabilities." *Disability & Society* 29 (6):863–876.

36 McIntosh, Tracey. 2005. "Maori identities: Fixed, fluid, forced." In *New Zealand identities: Departures and destinations*, edited by James H. Liu, Tim McCreanor, Tracey McIntosh and Teresia Teaiwa, 38–51. Wellington: Victoria University Press.

37 Patton, George C, Susan M Sawyer, John S Santelli, David A Ross, Rima Afifi, Nicholas B Allen, Monika Arora, Peter Azzopardi, Wendy Baldwin, and Christopher Bonell. 2016. "Our future: A Lancet commission on adolescent health and wellbeing." *The Lancet* 387 (10036):2423–2478.

38 Bottino, Sara, Mota Borges, Cássio Bottino, Caroline Gomez Regina, Aline Villa, Lobo Correia, and Wagner Silva Ribeiro. 2015. "Cyberbullying and adolescent mental health: Systematic review." *Cadernos de Saúde Pública* 31:463–475.

39 Dew, Kevin, Anthony Dowell, Deborah McLeod, Sunny Collings, and John Bushnell. 2005. ""This glorious twilight zone of uncertainty": Mental health consultations in general practice in New Zealand." *Social Science & Medicine* 61 (6):1189–1200.

40 Wodehouse, Pelham Grenville. 1963. *Stiff upper lip, Jeeves.* New York: Simon and Schuster.

41 Donald, Shane. 2018. "It's a colonial thing: New Zealand cultural identity and the use of 'colony' as a social category in intercultural communication." *New Zealand Studies in Applied Linguistics* 24 (1):5–17.

42 Ehrenreich, Barbara 2009. *Bright sided: How the relentless promotion of positive thinking has undermined America*: New York: Metropolitan Books.

43 Gable, Shelly L, and Jonathan Haidt. 2005. "What (and why) is positive psychology?" *Review of General Psychology* 9 (2):103–110.

44 Fleming, John, and Robert J Ledogar. 2008. "Resilience, an evolving concept: A review of literature relevant to Aboriginal research." *Pimatisiwin* 6 (2):7.

45 Jackson, Debra, Angela Firtko, and Michel Edenborough. 2007. "Personal resilience as a strategy for surviving and thriving in the face of workplace adversity: a literature review." *Journal of Avanced Nursing* 60 (1):1–9.

46 Waters, Lea. 2011. "A review of school-based positive psychology interventions." *The Educational and Developmental Psychologist* 28 (2):75–90.

47 McRobbie, Angela. 2007. "Top girls? Young women and the post-feminist sexual contract." *Cultural Studies* 21 (4–5):718–737.

48 Chowdhury, Nilima, Kerry Gibson, and Margaret Wetherell. 2020. "Polyphonies of depression: The relationship between voices-of-the-self in young professional women aka 'top girls'." *Health* 24 (6):773–790.

49 Perry, Felicity. 2015. "'Keeping it real': Tryhards, clones and youth discourses of authentic identity from Hollywood to high school." *Journal of Youth Studies* 18 (7):914–931.

50 American Psychiatric Association. 2013. *Diagnostic and statistical manual of mental disorders (DSM-5®)*. 5th ed. Arlington, VA: American Psychiatric Publishing.

51 World Health Organization. 2018. International classification of diseases for mortality and morbidity statistics (11th Revision). *World Health Organization.* Accessed 25February2021. Retrieved from https://icd.who.int/browse11/l-m/en.

52 Wakefield, Jerome C. 2016. "Diagnostic issues and controversies in DSM-5: Return of the false positives problem." *Annual Review of Clinical Psychology* 12:105–132.

53 Johnstone, Lucy, and Mary Boyle. 2019. "The power threat meaning framework: An alternative nondiagnostic conceptual system." *Journal of Humanistic Psychology* 1:18.
54 Rose, Diana, and Graham Thornicroft. 2010. "Service user perspectives on the impact of a mental illness diagnosis." *Epidemiology and Psychiatric Sciences* 19 (2):140–147.
55 Perkins, Amorette, Joseph Ridler, Daniel Browes, Guy Peryer, Caitlin Notley, and Corinna Hackmann. 2018. "Experiencing mental health diagnosis: A systematic review of service user, clinician, and carer perspectives across clinical settings." *The Lancet Psychiatry* 5 (9):747–764.
56 Wei, Yifeng, Jill A Hayden, Stan Kutcher, Austin Zygmunt, and Patrick McGrath. 2013. "The effectiveness of school mental health literacy programs to address knowledge, attitudes and help seeking among youth." *Early Intervention in Psychiatry* 7 (2):109–121.
57 Prout, H. Thompson. 2007. "Counseling and psychotherapy with children and adolescents: Historical, developmental, integrative and effectiveness perspectives." In *Counseling and psychotherapy with children and adolescents: Theory and practice for school and clinical settings*, edited byH Thompson Prout and Douglas T Brown, 1–31. Hoboken, New Jersey: John Wiley & Sons.
58 Kelly, Peter. 2000. "The dangerousness of youth-at-risk: The possibilities of surveillance and intervention in uncertain times." *Journal of Adolescence* 23 (4):463–476.
59 Hollings, James. 2013. "Reporting suicide in New Zealand: Time to end censorship." *Pacific Journalism Review* 19 (2):136–155.
60 Rickwood, Debra, Frank P Deane, Coralie J Wilson, and Joseph Ciarrochi. 2005. "Young people's help-seeking for mental health problems." *Australian e-journal for the Advancement of Mental health* 4 (3):218–251.
61 Marcia, James E. 1980. "Identity in adolescence." *Handbook of Adolescent Psychology* 9 (11):159–187.
62 Erikson, Erik H. 1968. *Identity: Youth and crisis.* New York: WW Norton & Company.
63 Bamberg, Michael, Anna De Fina, and Deborah Schiffrin. 2011. "Discourse and Identity Construction." In *Handbook of identity theory and research*, edited by Seth J Schwartz, Koen Luyckx and Vivian L Vignoles, 177–199. New York, NY: Springer New York.
64 Bussey, Kay. 2011. "Gender identity development." In *Handbook of identity theory and research*, edited by Seth J Schwartz, Koen Luyckx and Vivian L Vignoles, 603–628. New York, NY: Springer New York.
65 Gavey, Nicola. 2012. "Beyond "empowerment"? Sexuality in a sexist world." *Sex Roles* 66 (11–12):718–724.
66 Leit, Richard A, James J Gray, and Harrison G Pope Jr. 2002. "The media's representation of the ideal male body: A cause for muscle dysmorphia?" *International Journal of Eating Disorders* 31 (3):334–338.
67 Andermann, Lisa. 2010. "Culture and the social construction of gender: Mapping the intersection with mental health." *International Review of Psychiatry* 22 (5):501–512.
68 Lafrance, Michelle N, and Suzanne McKenzie-Mohr. 2013. "The DSM and its lure of legitimacy." *Feminism & Psychology* 23 (1):119–140.
69 Cleary, Anne. 2012. "Suicidal action, emotional expression, and the performance of masculinities." *Social Science & Medicine* 74 (4):498–505.

70 McDermott, Elizabeth, and Katrina Roen. 2016. *Queer youth, suicide and self-harm: Troubled subjects, troubling norms.* Houndmills, UK: Palgrave Nacmillan.
71 Nilan, Pam, and Carles Feixa. 2006. *Global youth?: Hybrid identities, plural worlds.* New York: Routledge.
72 Bates, Adam, Trish Hobman, and Beth T Bell. 2020. "Let me do what i please with it... Don't decide my identity for me: LGBTQ+ youth experiences of social media in narrative identity development." *Journal of Adolescent Research* 35 (1):51–83.
73 Woodgate, Roberta L, Christine Ateah, and Loretta Secco. 2008. "Living in a world of our own: The experience of parents who have a child with autism." *Qualitative Health Research* 18 (8):1075–1083.
74 Sickel, Amy E, Jason D Seacat, and Nina A Nabors. 2014. "Mental health stigma update: A review of consequences." *Advances in Mental Health* 12 (3):202–215.
75 Rüsch, Nicolas, Matthias C Angermeyer, and Patrick W Corrigan. 2005. "Mental illness stigma: Concepts, consequences, and initiatives to reduce stigma." *European Psychiatry* 20 (8):529–539.
76 Nordt, Carlos, Wulf Rössler, and Christoph Lauber. 2006. "Attitudes of mental health professionals toward people with schizophrenia and major depression." *Schizophrenia Bulletin* 32 (4):709–714.
77 Corrigan, Patrick W, Amy C Watson, and Leah Barr. 2006. "The self–stigma of mental illness: Implications for self–esteem and self–efficacy." *Journal of Social and Clinical Psychology* 25 (8):875–884.
78 Hartman, Leah I, Natalie M Michel, Ariella Winter, Rebecca E Young, Gordon L Flett, and Joel O Goldberg. 2013. "Self-stigma of mental illness in high school youth." *Canadian Journal of School Psychology* 28 (1):28–42.
79 Naslund, JA, KA Aschbrenner, LA Marsch, and SJ Bartels. 2016. "The future of mental health care: Peer-to-peer support and social media." *Epidemiology and Psychiatric Sciences* 25 (2):113–122.
80 Parsloe, Sarah M. 2015. "Discourses of disability, narratives of community: Reclaiming an autistic identity online." *Journal of Applied Communication Research* 43 (3):336–356.
81 Yeshua-Katz, Daphna. 2015. "Online stigma resistance in the pro-ana community." *Qualitative Health Research* 25 (10):1347–1358.
82 Lynch, Johanna M., Deborah A. Askew, Geoffrey K. Mitchell, and Kelsey L. Hegarty. 2012. "Beyond symptoms: Defining primary care mental health clinical assessment priorities, content and process". *Social Science & Medicine* 74 (2):143–149.
83 APA Presidential Task Force on Evidence-Based Practice. 2006. "Evidence-based practice in psychology." *American Psychologist* 61 (4):271–285. doi: 10.1037/0003-066x.61.4.271.
84 Spear, Hila J, and Pamela Kulbok. 2004. "Autonomy and adolescence: A concept analysis." *Public Health Nursing* 21 (2):144–152.
85 Bandura, Albert. 2006. "Toward a psychology of human agency." *Perspectives on Psychological Science* 1 (2):164–180.
86 Bruner, Jerome. 1990. *Acts of meaning.* Cambridge, MA, US: Harvard University Press.
87 LeMoyne, Terri, and Tom Buchanan. 2011. "Does "hovering" matter? Helicopter parenting and its effect on well-being." *Sociological Spectrum* 31 (4):399–418.

88 Thompson, Richard, Laura J Proctor, Diana J English, Howard Dubowitz, Subasri Narasimhan, and Mark D Everson. 2012. "Suicidal ideation in adolescence: Examining the role of recent adverse experiences." *Journal of Adolescence* 35 (1):175–186.

89 Aluede, Oyaziwo, Fajoju Adeleke, Don Omoike, and Justina Afen-Akpaida. 2008. "A review of the extent, nature, characteristics and effects of bullying behaviour in schools." *Journal of Instructional Psychology* 35 (2):151.

90 Alsop, Ruth, Mette Bertelsen, and Jeremy Holland. 2006. *Empowerment in practice: From analysis to implementation.* Washington D.C: The World Bank.

91 Kwon, Soo Ah. 2018. "The politics of global youth participation." *Journal of Youth Studies* 22 (7):926–940.

92 Duncan, Rony E, Annette C Hall, and Ann Knowles. 2015. "Ethical dilemmas of confidentiality with adolescent clients: Case studies from psychologists." *Ethics & Behavior* 25 (3):197–221.

93 Nichols, Michael P, and Richard C Schwartz. 2007. *The essentials of family therapy.* 3rd ed. Boston: Pearson/Allyn & Bacon.

94 Pitama, Suzanne G, Simon T Bennett, Waikaremoana Waitoki, Tracy N Haitanai, Hukarere Valentine, John Pahina, Joanne E Taylor, Natasha Tassell-Matamua, Luke Rowe, and Lutz Beckerti. 2017. "A proposed Hauora Maori clinical guide for psychologists: Using the Hui process and Meihana model in clinical assessment and formulation." *New Zealand Journal of Psychology* 46 (3):7.

95 Read, John, Claire Cartwright, and Kerry Gibson. 2014. "Adverse emotional and interpersonal effects reported by 1829 New Zealanders while taking antidepressants". *Psychiatry Research* 216 (1):67–73.

96 Block, Azadeh Masalehdan, and Catherine G Greeno. 2011. "Examining outpatient treatment dropout in adolescents: A literature review." *Child and Adolescent Social Work Journal* 28 (5):393–420.

97 Beutler, Larry E, Carla Moleiro, and Hani Talebi. 2002. "Resistance in psychotherapy: What conclusions are supported by research." *Journal of Clinical Psychology* 58 (2):207–217.

98 Sparks, Jacqueline A. 2002. "Taking a stand: An adolescent girl's resistance to medication." *Journal of Marital and Family Therapy* 28 (1):27–38.

99 Miller, Scott D, Barry L Duncan, Jeb Brown, Ryan Sorrell, and Mary Beth Chalk. 2006. "Using formal client feedback to improve retention and outcome: Making ongoing, real-time assessment feasible." *Journal of Brief Therapy* 5 (1):5–22.

100 Binder, Per-Einar, Christian Moltu, Didrik Hummelsund, Solfrid Henden Sagen, and Helge Holgersen. 2011. "Meeting an adult ally on the way out into the world: Adolescent patients' experiences of useful psychotherapeutic ways of working at an age when independence really matters." *Psychotherapy Research* 21 (5):554–566.

101 Sauter, Floor M, David Heyne, and P Michiel Westenberg. 2009. "Cognitive behavior therapy for anxious adolescents: Developmental influences on treatment design and delivery." *Clinical Child and Family Psychology Review* 12 (4):310–335.

102 Courtois, Christine A, and Julian D Ford. 2013. *Treatment of complex trauma: A sequenced, relationship-based approach.* New York: Guilford Press.

103 Ito, Mizuko, Heather Horst, Matteo Bittanti, Danah Boyd, Becky Herr- Stephenson, Patricia G Lange, CJ Pascoe, and Laura Robinson. 2008. *Living*

and learning with new media: summary of findings from the digital youth project. Chicago, Illinois: John D. and Catherine T. MacArthur Foundation.

104 Cohen, Sheldon, and Thomas A Wills. 1985. "Stress, social support, and the buffering hypothesis." *Psychological Bulletin* 98 (2):310.

105 Lambert, Michael J, and Dean E Barley. 2001. "Research summary on the therapeutic relationship and psychotherapy outcome." *Psychotherapy: Theory, Research, Practice, Training* 38 (4):357–361.

106 Ask, Kristine, and Crystal Abidin. 2018. "My life is a mess: Self-deprecating relatability and collective identities in the memification of student issues." *Information, Communication & Society* 21 (6):834–850.

107 Stanton-Salazar, Ricardo D, and Stephanie Urso Spina. 2005. "Adolescent peer networks as a context for social and emotional support." *Youth & Society* 36 (4):379–417.

108 Rickwood, Debra, Frank P Deane, and Coralie J Wilson. 2007. "When and how do young people seek professional help for mental health problems?" *Medical Journal of Australia*187 (7 Suppl): S35–S39.

109 Castonguay, Louis G, Michael J Constantino, and Martin Grosse Holtforth. 2006. "The working alliance: Where are we and where should we go?" *Psychotherapy: Theory, Research, Practice, Training* 43 (3):271.

110 Palitsky, Daniel, Natalie Mota, Tracie O Afifi, A Craig Downs, and Jitender Sareen. 2013. "The association between adult attachment style, mental disorders, and suicidality: Findings from a population-based study". *The Journal of Nervous and Mental Disease* 201 (7):579–586.

111 Binnie, James. 2015. "Do you want therapy with that? A critical account of working within IAPT." *Mental Health Review Journal* 20 (2):79–83.

112 Jamieson, Kathleen Hall, and Daniel Romer. 2005. "A call to action on adolescent mental health." In *Treating and Preventing Adolescent Mental Health Disorders: What We Know and What We Don't Know*, edited by Edna B Foa, Dwight L. Evans, Raquel E Gur, Herbert Hendin, Charles P. O'Brien, Martin EP Seligman and B. Timothy Walsh, 598–617. New York: Oxford University Press.

113 Peterson, Zoë D. 2002. "More than a mirror: The ethics of therapist self-disclosure." *Psychotherapy: Theory, Research, Practice, Training* 39 (1):21–31.

114 Fox, Claire L, and Ian Butler. 2007. "'If you don't want to tell anyone else you can tell her': Young people's views on school counselling." *British Journal of Guidance & Counselling* 35 (1):97–114.

115 Gulliver, Amelia, Kathleen M Griffiths, and Helen Christensen. 2010. "Perceived barriers and facilitators to mental health help-seeking in young people: A systematic review." *BMC Psychiatry* 10 (1):1–9.

116 Ramsden, Edmund. 2019. "Designing for mental health: Psychiatry, psychology and the architectural study project." In *Preventing mental illness: Past, present and future*, edited by Despo Kritsotaki, Vicky Long and Matthew Smith, 209–235. Cham, Switzerland: Palgrave Macmillan.

117 West, Monique, Glenn Melvin, Francis McNamara, and Michael Gordon. 2017. "An evaluation of the use and efficacy of a sensory room within an adolescent psychiatric inpatient unit." *Australian Occupational Therapy Journal* 64 (3):253–263.

118 Gray, Anne. 1994. *An introduction to the therapeutic frame.* London: Routledge.

119 Radez, Jerica, Tessa Reardon, Cathy Creswell, Peter J Lawrence, Georgina Evdoka-Burton, and Polly Waite. 2020. "Why do children and adolescents (not)

seek and access professional help for their mental health problems? A systematic review of quantitative and qualitative studies." *European Child & Adolescent Psychiatry* 30: 1–29.

120 Jorm, Anthony F, Annemarie Wright, and Amy J Morgan. 2007. "Where to seek help for a mental disorder?" *Medical Journal of Australia* 187 (10):556–560.

121 Summerhurst, Carolyn, Michael Wammes, Andrew Wrath, and Elizabeth Osuch. 2017. "Youth perspectives on the mental health treatment process: What helps, what hinders?" *Community Mental Health Journal* 53 (1):72–78.

122 Paterson, Ron, Mason Durie, Barbara Disley, Dean Rangihuna, Jemaima Sipaea Tiatia-Seath, and Josiah Tualamali'i. 2018. *He Ara Oranga: Report of the government inquiry into mental health and addiction.* Wellington: New Zealand Government.

123 Lamsal, Ramesh, Carol A Stalker, Cheryl-Anne Cait, Manuel Riemer, and Susan Horton. 2017. "Cost-effectiveness analysis of single-session walk-in counselling." *Journal of Mental Health* 27 (6):560–566.

124 Reese, Robert J, Collie W Conoley, and Daniel F Brossart. 2002. "Effectiveness of telephone counseling: A field-based investigation." *Journal of counseling Psychology* 49 (2):233.

125 Gibson, Kerry, and Claire Cartwright. 2014. "Young people's experiences of mobile phone text counselling: Balancing connection and control." *Children and Youth Services Review* 43:96–104.

126 Uhlhaas, Peter, and John Torous. 2019. "Digital tools for youth mental health." *NPJ Digital Medicine* 2:104.

127 Prensky, Marc. 2001. "Digital natives, digital immigrants part 1." *On the Horizon* 9 (5):1–6.

128 Helsper, Ellen Johanna, and Rebecca Eynon. 2010. "Digital natives: Where is the evidence?" *British Educational Research Journal* 36 (3):503–520.

129 . Anderson, Monica, and Jingjing Jiang. 2018. "Teens, social media & technology." *Pew Research Center* 1–19. Accessed 25 February 2021. Retrieved from https://assets.pewresearch.org/wp-content/uploads/sites/14/2018/05/31102617/PI_2018.05.31_TeensTech_FINAL.pdf.

130 Anderson Katie, Elson. 2020. "Getting acquainted with social networks and apps: It is time to talk about TikTok." *Library Hi Tech News* 37 (4):7–12.

131 O'Reilly, Michelle, Nisha Dogra, Natasha Whiteman, Jason Hughes, Seyda Eruyar, and Paul Reilly. 2018. "Is social media bad for mental health and wellbeing? Exploring the perspectives of adolescents." *Clinical Child Psychology and Psychiatry* 23 (4):601–613.

132 McGlynn, Clare, Kelly Johnson, Erika Rackley, Nicola Henry, Nicola Gavey, Asher Flynn, and Anastasia Powell. 2020. "'It's torture for the soul': The harms of image based sexual abuse." *Social & Legal Studies* 1–22. 10.1177/0964663920965748

133 Craig, Wendy, Meyran Boniel-Nissim, Nathan King, Sophie D Walsh, Maartje Boer, Peter D Donnelly, Yossi Harel-Fisch, Marta Malinowska-Cieślik, Margarida Gaspar de Matos, and Alina Cosma. 2020. "Social media use and cyber-bullying: A cross-national analysis of young people in 42 countries." *Journal of Adolescent Health* 66 (6):S100–S108.

134 Kowalski, Robin M, and Susan P Limber. 2007. "Electronic bullying among middle school students." *Journal of Adolescent Health* 41 (6):S22–S30.

135 Jorgenson, Alicia Grattan, Ray Chih-Jui Hsiao, and Cheng-Fang Yen. 2016. "Internet addiction and other behavioral addictions." *Child and Adolescent Psychiatric Clinics* 25 (3):509–520.

136 Weinstein, Aviv, and Michel Lejoyeux. 2010. "Internet addiction or excessive internet use." *The American Journal of Drug and Alcohol Abuse* 36 (5):277–283.

137 Levy, Neil. 2013. "Addiction is not a brain disease (and it matters)." *Frontiers in Psychiatry* 4 (24):1–7.

138 Iskender, Murat. 2018. "Investigation of the effects of social self-confidence, social loneliness and family emotional loneliness variables on internet addiction." *Malaysian Online Journal of Educational Technology* 6 (3):1–10.

139 Wilson, Sara. 2020. "The era of antisocial social media." *Harvard Business Review*. Accessed 22 February 2021. Retrieved from https://hbr.org/2020/02/the-eraof-antisocial-social-media.

140 Cohen, Hart. 2000. "Revisiting McLuhan." *Media International Australia, Incorporating Culture & Policy* (94):5–12.

141 . Orlowski, Jeff. 2020. *The social dilemma. Netflix*. Retrieved from https://www.netflix.com/nz/title/81254224.

142 Clarke, Aleisha M, Tuuli Kuosmanen, and Margaret M Barry. 2015. "A systematic review of online youth mental health promotion and prevention interventions." *Journal of Youth and Adolescence* 44 (1):90–113.

143 Rickwood, Debra J. 2011. "Promoting youth mental health: Priorities for policy from an Australian perspective." *Early Intervention in Psychiatry* 5:40–45.

144 Kelly, Claire M, Anthony F Jorm, and Annemarie Wright. 2007. "Improving mental health literacy as a strategy to facilitate early intervention for mental disorders." *Medical Journal of Australia* 187 (S7):S26–S30.

145 Swar, Bobby, Tahir Hameed, and Iris Reychav. 2017. "Information overload, psychological ill-being, and behavioral intention to continue online healthcare information search." *Computers in Human Behavior* 70: 416–425.

146 Morahan-Martin, Janet, and Colleen D Anderson. 2000. "Information and misinformation online: Recommendations for facilitating accurate mental health information retrieval and evaluation." *CyberPsychology & Behavior* 3 (5):731–746.

147 Parekh, Natasha, and William H. Shrank. 2018. "Dangers and opportunities of direct-to-consumer advertising." *Journal of General Internal Medicine* 33 (5):586–587.

148 Merry, Sally N, Karolina Stasiak, Matthew Shepherd, Chris Frampton, Theresa Fleming, and Mathijs F G Lucassen. 2012. "The effectiveness of SPARX, a computerised self help intervention for adolescents seeking help for depression: Randomised controlled non-inferiority trial." *British Medical Journal* 344:1–16.

149 Anthes, Emily. 2016. "Mental health: There's an app for that." *Nature News* 532 (7597):20–23.

150 Ersahin, Zehra, and Terry Hanley. 2017. "Using text-based synchronous chat to offer therapeutic support to students: A systematic review of the research literature." *Health Education Journal* 76 (5):531–543.

151 Suler, John. 2004. "The online disinhibition effect." *Cyberpsychology & Behavior* 7 (3):321–326.

152 Alleman, James R. 2002. "Online counseling: The Internet and mental health treatment." *Psychotherapy: Theory, Research, Practice, Training* 39 (2):199.

153 Lewis, Stephen P, and Yukari Seko. 2016. "A double-edged sword: A review of benefits and risks of online nonsuicidal self-injury activities." *Journal of Clinical Psychology* 72 (3):249–262.

154 Chorpita, Bruce F, Eric L Daleiden, Chad Ebesutani, John Young, Kimberly D Becker, Brad J Nakamura, Lisa Phillips, Alyssa Ward, Roxanna Lynch, and Lindsay Trent. 2011. "Evidence-based treatments for children and adolescents: An updated review of indicators of efficacy and effectiveness." *Clinical Psychology: Science and Practice* 18 (2):154–172.

155 Harris, Maxine, and Roger D Fallot. 2009. *Creating cultures of trauma-informed care (CCTIC): A self-assessment and planning protocol.* Washington D.C.: Community Connections.

156 Hetrick, Sarah E, Alan P Bailey, Kirsten E Smith, Ashok Malla, Steve Mathias, Swaran P Singh, Aileen O'Reilly, Swapna K Verma, Laelia Benoit, and Theresa M Fleming. 2017. "Integrated (one-stop shop) youth health care: Best available evidence and future directions." *Medical Journal of Australia* 207 (S10):S5–S18.

157 McGorry, Patrick, Jason Trethowan, and Debra Rickwood. 2019. "Creating headspace for integrated youth mental health care." *World Psychiatry* 18 (2):140.

158 Garrett, Susan, Susan Pullon, Sonya Morgan, and Eileen McKinlay. 2020. "Collaborative care in 'youth one stop shops' in New Zealand: Hidden, time consuming, essential." *Journal of Child Health Care* 24 (2):180–194.

159 Burns, Jane M, Emma Birrell, Marie Bismark, Jane Pirkis, Tracey A Davenport, Ian B Hickie, Melissa K Weinberg, and Louise A Ellis. 2016. "The role of technology in Australian youth mental health reform." *Australian Health Review* 40 (5):584–590.

160 Gindidis, Simone, Sandra E Stewart, and John Roodenburg. 2020. "Adolescent experiences of app-integrated therapy." *The Educational and Developmental Psychologist* 37 (1):20–29.

161 Live For Tomorrow. 2019. Live For Tomorrow. October 2019 Report Auckland, New Zealand.

162 Thorn, Pinar, Nicole TM Hill, Michelle Lamblin, Zoe Teh, Rikki Battersby-Coulter, Simon Rice, Sarah Bendall, Kerry L Gibson, Summer May Finlay, and Ryan Blandon. 2020. "Developing a suicide prevention social media campaign with young people (The #Chatsafe project): Co-design approach." *JMIR Mental Health* 7 (5):e17520.

163 Faithfull, Sarah, Lisa Brophy, Kerryn Pennell, and Magenta B Simmons. 2019. "Barriers and enablers to meaningful youth participation in mental health research: Qualitative interviews with youth mental health researchers." *Journal of Mental Health* 28 (1):56–63.

164 Ali, Kathina, Louise Farrer, Amelia Gulliver, and Kathleen M Griffiths. 2015. "Online peer-to-peer support for young people with mental health problems: A systematic review." *JMIR* 2 (2):e19.

165 Barton, Jessica, and Joanna Henderson. 2016. "Peer support and youth recovery: A brief review of the theoretical underpinnings and evidence." *Canadian Journal of Family and Youth/Le Journal Canadien de Famille et de la Jeunesse* 8 (1):1–17.

166 Arthur, Nancy, ed. 2019. *Counselling in cultural contexts: Identities and social justice.* Cham: Springer.

167 Bolton, Julie. 2017. "The ethical issues which must be addressed in online counselling." *Australian Counselling Research Journal* 11 (1):1–15.

Index

For Product Safety Concerns and Information please contact our EU
representative GPSR@taylorandfrancis.com
Taylor & Francis Verlag GmbH, Kaufingerstraße 24, 80331 München, Germany

www.ingramcontent.com/pod-product-compliance
Lightning Source LLC
Chambersburg PA
CBHW070342270326
41926CB00017B/3951

* 9 7 8 0 3 6 7 3 3 8 5 9 6 *